Become a Popcorn Genius

Kelli and Frank DeMaio

GPP

Great Point Publishing, LLC

Gloversville, NY

Become a Popcorn Genius
Kelli and Frank DeMaio

DISCLAIMER:
The advice contained in this material might not be suitable for everyone. The information presented is based on the author's experience and research and in no way guarantees that the reader will achieve any specific set of results by applying the ideas detailed on the following pages. It is the full responsibility of the reader to evaluate the suitability of the ideas, tactics, and strategies discussed to their own individual situation and business. In particular, the author accepts no responsibility for the results achieved by applying these strategies. The author particularly disclaims any liability, loss, or risk taken by individuals who directly or indirectly act on contained on the information contained herein. The author believes that the advice presented here is sound, but readers cannot hold him responsible for either the actions they take, or the results of those actions.

Cover Design By: Kara DeMaio
Book design by: Great Point Publishing LLC

To order additional copies of this title, contact your favorite local bookstore or visit *www.greatpointpublishing.com*

Paperback ISBN: 978-1-955334-99-0

Printed in the United States of America

Published by: ***Great Point Publishing, LLC.***
Gloversville, NY

Dedication.

This book is dedicated to our sons Luca and Frankie.

We love you!

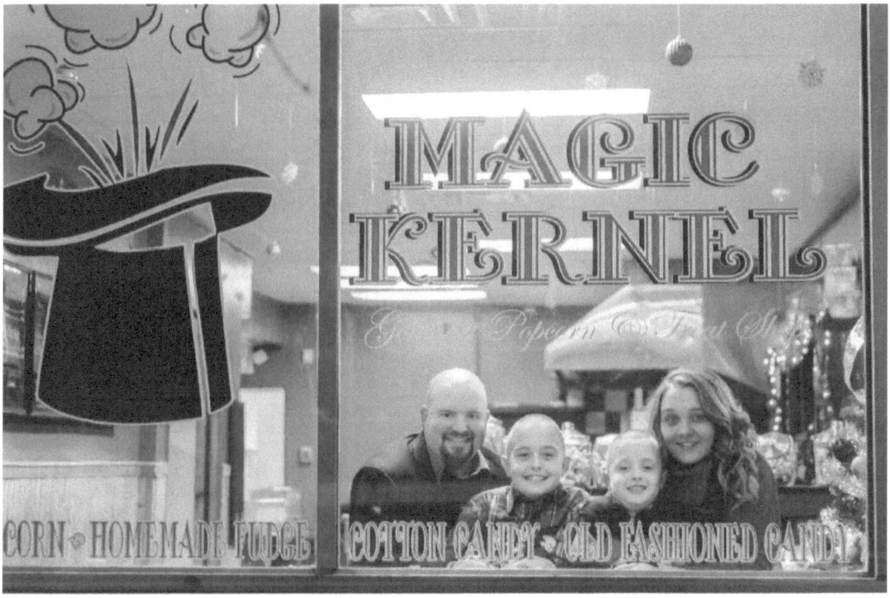

Frank, Luca, Frankie, and Kelli at The Magic Kernel, their gourmet popcorn shop in Johnstown, NY.
December 7, 2013

Thanks, and Acknowledgements

A huge & heartfelt thank you to our family and friends for always supporting us through our adventures.

And especially to our parents, Cubby & Mary Jo, Delores & Fred, and Tony.... Thank you for teaching us to dream big and work hard. But most importantly for showing & instilling in us our most valued lesson

... FAMILY FIRST.

Table of Contents

Become a Popcorn Genius

Chapter 1

Our Story

Hi! We are Kelli and Frank, a husband-and-wife team who have been married for over 22 years, and WE LOVE popcorn. Our popcorn life includes making new popcorn recipes, sharing it with friends, and of course eating it. We love popcorn so much that a few years back, we took that love for our favorite treat and turned it into our livelihood.

We are not alone, but just two of the over 230 million Americans that consumed a portion of 14 billion quarts of popcorn in 2020. Not only is that number mind boggling but it is growing. In fact, $9.86 billion was generated in the popcorn industry in 2020 and is projected to grow to $18.82 billion by 2031.

Our story in making and selling popcorn began one night when we were out to dinner where somehow during our conversation one of us jokingly said it would be so much fun to own a gourmet popcorn shop. The conversation was full of ideas. We talked about all of the different flavors of popcorn we could make, types of old-fashioned candy we could sell, flavors of homemade fudge we could make, and so much more. It may have been a crazy idea, but that did not stop us from imagining it all. Both of us were so excited over the possibility that we even started drawing out how the shop would look.

The next day that excitement turned to research with the first step of learning all it would take for us to make this happen. We researched equipment, products, types of permits needed, and even locations. It was not very long after that we came up with a name, The Magic Kernel. Our logo was a top hat that was turned upside down with popcorn popping out of the hat. There were so many things to think about, and we were unsure of what to do first. There was a large upfront cost with the equipment being extremely expensive. We knew that we needed a popper and a caramelizer, but we also wanted a copper kettle to be able to make old fashioned caramel corn. The desire to want the copper kettle was inspired from a family weekend getaway. We had watched someone make caramel corn in a cooper kettle in Syracuse, NY at a shop we had visited. Quickly, we started to realize just how expensive starting this business was going to be. With the equipment and all the incidentals such as measuring cups, utensils, trays, storage containers, buckets, cooling trays, tables, etc., the costs were really going up there. We were not giving up though; we were determined to find a way to make it happen.

the MAGIC KERNEL

Gourmet Popcorn

A few weeks had passed, and an ad popped up in the classifieds. Someone had listed a large amount of gourmet popcorn equipment for sale. It was like a sign! We were in such disbelief because this was not a typical listing you would see in the classified. This seemed like such a rare opportunity that we decided to jump at the chance. We contacted the seller of the equipment and found out that they had a few gourmet popcorn locations but closed one down recently. All of their equipment was in a storage unit, and he was ready to sell. He sent what pictures he had as he was about three hours away. Based on what we saw, we were in. As the equipment came to fruition, right on cue, a location popped up on our radar. Another sign we could not ignore. We set up a meeting to look at the building, rented a box truck, and set a date to pick up the equipment.

Even though the building was currently undergoing some renovations, it was exactly what we were looking for. We signed a lease and secured the location. A couple of days later we picked up the box truck, and along with our brother-in-law and a family friend we made the 3-hour drive to pick up the equipment. When we got there, we were blown away when he lifted the storage locker door. There was so much equipment packed in that small space. The first thing we saw was a big 20oz theater-style popcorn popper, and as we started to unload the unit, the other equipment started to come into view. There was a 5-gallon caramelizer, a copper kettle, cooling trays, containers, counters and shelving units, signage, spoons, knives, thermometers, food safe buckets, measuring cups, stainless steel trays, utensils, a commercial hot water heater, and a ton more. He even included some recipes for us to get started. We packed that truck chock full and headed home.

We unloaded all of our equipment into our garage while we waited for renovations to be completed. In the meantime, we worked on the shop in our free time. We worked on signage, permits, paint, built-in counters, and a lot more. After a few weeks and with the help and support of our family and friends, the shop was all set up. The next item on our checklist was placing our first food order for all the products and ingredients. We had never made most of the flavor ideas we had come up with, but we knew we would figure it out.

We were so excited that everything was coming together that we decided to open on the night of the town's holiday parade. We had gotten ahead of ourselves for sure, as the parade was only four days after our first food order would arrive. No pressure, right?

Even though we purchased all the right equipment, the one thing we didn't get was training. We never made gourmet popcorn or flavored popcorn in our lives, and we had four days to figure out how to make more than 24 flavors. The pressure started to sink in, but we are not the type to back down from a challenge, so we got to work.

Right off the bat we ran into a problem with the automatic oil dispenser that was attached to the popper. We had to figure out how to get the heating element into a solid 5-gallon pail of butter coconut oil. The simplest solution (because we had no idea what we were doing) was to simply carve a hole. So, we found a giant machete like cheese knife and started carving a hole right down the middle for the heating element to fit into. Once that was set, the pump needed to be calibrated for our size machine. After some trial and error, we started to pop some plain popcorn. This was only the first step. We popped gallons of plain popcorn knowing we needed to flavor it.

The first thing we wanted to do was to try to use the caramelizer. This machine is basically a large stainless-steel pot that heats up on its own and has a stirring mechanism built it. It's used to put candy coatings on popcorn. Not all of the equipment had come with instructions, and we had tried to find whatever information we could prior to using the machine. The first few batches came out with either no flavor at all or burnt with a dark color. It took us a while to realize that we added the flavoring too early in the process and all the flavor burned off. We also realized we were heating the mixture too long and not to the right temperature. After a lot of trial and error, we were finally getting the mixtures and recipes right. The presentation was important to us, so nice bright colors for our popcorn were important and we didn't stop practicing until we got it perfect.

Next, we wanted to make caramel corn. The equipment we purchased had a large copper kettle that sat on an electric heating unit powered by light bulbs. Yes, you read that right, light bulbs! We thought back to that time when we visited the caramel corn shop in Syracuse and started to get excited. We had to get the process just right which included bringing the caramel mixture just to the right temperature. If the right temperature isn't achieved, either too much or too little the corn would come out drab, burned, or soggy. The secret recipe we developed which included all homemade ingredients like butter, brown sugar, and other ingredients is terrific. On top of that, we were able to get the combination of heat and time just right to create a nice shiny, wonderfully flavored caramel corn which to this day we are proud of.

After getting the sweet flavors figured out, it was time to tackle the savory flavors. This was so much easier. You literally pop the corn and then shake it with seasoning. The trial-and-error part of this is figuring out the perfect amount of seasoning and how to get the mix to stick to the popcorn. Once we realized that the seasoning sticks better to fresh hot popcorn and adjusted the seasonings, everything was turning out great.

We didn't get much sleep over the next couple days. All of the testing and perfecting resulted in gallons and gallons of popcorn being thrown away. We were getting more confident and with only one day away from our opening we had a lot of work to do. As excited as we were we were equally nervous and overwhelmed. We needed to get popping. We made over 300 gallons of popcorn consisting of 25 different flavors, just in preparation for opening day. That amount does not include the popcorn we threw out.

We filled our display shelves with all the flavors and creations. We made kettle corn, caramel corn, butter, salt and vinegar, sour cream and chive, bacon and cheese, cheddar cheese, white cheddar cheese, chocolate covered caramel corn, watermelon, green apple, lemon, orange, blue raspberry, black cherry, grape, birthday cake, s'mores, butter toffee crunch, chocolate, ranch, BBQ, garlic parm, hot and spicy, pizza, and more.

Our goal was to open in time for the holiday parade and we did it! On the night of the parade, the streets were filled with people. The line for the shop went down the entire block and opening night was a huge success.

The number of flavors we offered our customers gave us a sense of pride. We could boast over 25 flavors of gourmet popcorn, and that didn't even include the combo flavors. As a customer you could get any combination of our flavors that you wanted. That included mixing caramel corn with cheddar corn or green apple popcorn. Mixing pizza popcorn and ranch popcorn, or sour cream and chive popcorn with bacon and cheese popcorn. Our customers would come in and make up their own creative combinations which made it a fun environment.

The best thing about owning and running a popcorn shop is that every customer that comes in is just in a great mood. I mean how could you not be in a great mood buying popcorn? Our customers were loyal, amazing, and wonderfully supportive people. We knew our regular customers' favorite flavors and some even joined the popcorn club where you could bring your 2-gallon tin back in for discounted refills.

The success never ended, and we continued to thrive. Owning the shop was so much fun. Friends and family would stop in to visit and to help us out. A community of people formed on its own, all revolving around popcorn. While it was a lot of work, it was also a lot of fun, which we enjoyed.

Unfortunately, our family experienced some devastating losses. Even though we had the support of the community, it was extremely impactful to our family. After taking stock in our life, we decided it was time to spend more time with our family and less time running the shop. We made a hard decision to close the shop down "temporarily". By 'temporarily', we told ourselves we would open back up later in life. To that end we put all of our equipment in storage so we could open our shop up again one day. While we were sad to close the shop, we know we made the right decision because family always comes first.

Even though we closed the shop, that didn't mean we stopped loving, popping, and sharing popcorn.

Our love of watching others enjoy our popcorn has never stopped or even slowed down as we continue to make all kinds of flavors to this day.

We made so many different flavor combinations over the years for customers. Even now, when we see people around town, we remember them by the popcorn flavor they always came in and got. Over the years we have even helped others make their own favorite popcorn creations.

This includes consulting with new businesses to help them get their doors opened in the gourmet popcorn world. We started a YouTube channel under the name Popcorn Genius to teach others how to make popcorn. And in 2024, we wrote our first book on popcorn, the one that you're reading now, and we absolutely can't wait to teach you and help you Become a Popcorn Genius!

Here are some of the things that you'll learn about in the following chapters.

You'll learn about the history and science of popping corn, and lots of fun facts! You'll read about health information of popcorn, and specific tips such as the perfect temperature to cook popcorn, and the perfect moisture content. Then we get to teach you some of our favorite popcorn recipes, including specific ingredients such as what type of oil to use and the difference between different popcorn kernels, so you can make the best popcorn possible for your friends and family!

We hope that sounds as much fun to you as it does to us!

Like we said earlier, we LOVE popcorn. We love watching others enjoy our popcorn; and now we can't wait to teach you more. Let's get poppin!

Chapter 2

The History of Popcorn

Popcorn, a cherished snack that has stood the test of time and crossed cultural boundaries, boasts a rich history spanning thousands of years. It all started in the ancient Americas, and now people from every corner of the world savor popcorn. Ready for a quick and fun journey through popcorn's captivating history? We'll explore its ancient roots, cultural significance, and how it continues to be a beloved snack in today's world.

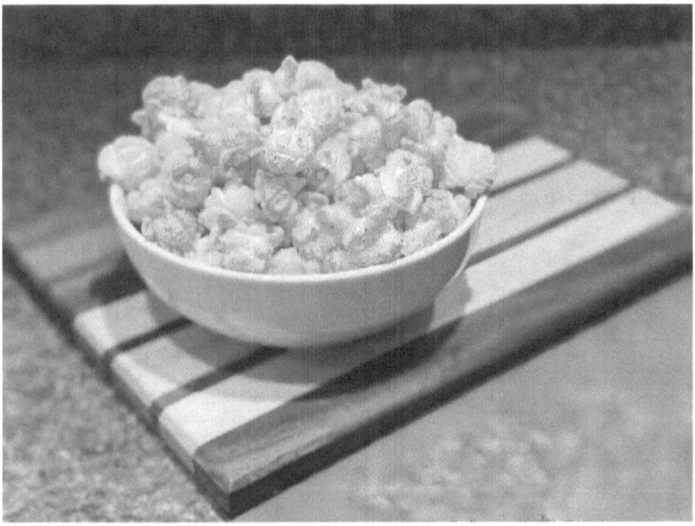

Popcorn has been popping since ancient times, with evidence of its existence in the Americas dating back thousands of years. This magical puffed-up corn has held various roles in different cultures, from being a nutritious food option to a part of religious ceremonies or even a decorative element. As the world grew more interconnected, popcorn crossed oceans and started mingling with the culinary traditions of numerous cultures.

Fast forward to today, and popcorn is practically the ultimate symbol of fun and entertainment. It's the go-to munchie for movie theaters, sports events, and cozy family nights. Our favorite crunchy and airy treat has evolved into a versatile snack, boasting a wide array of flavors and styles to satisfy every craving. Plus, popcorn has popped its way into the global culinary scene, with countries and cultures worldwide adding their own unique twists to this scrumptious snack.

The ongoing allure of popcorn can be credited to its captivating history, cultural significance, and adaptable nature. From its ancient roots in the Americas to its current status as a global snack sensation, popcorn has continued to be a comforting and constant presence in people's lives. As we delve deeper into the history of popcorn in the following sections, we hope you'll join us on this tasty journey through time and perhaps develop a new appreciation for this ageless treat.

Unearthing Popcorn's Ancient Roots

Popcorn's fascinating history starts with archaeological findings in Mexico, Peru, and the United States. These remnants of this ancient snack provide invaluable insights into its usage by ancient civilizations. In Mexico, the Bat Cave, located in the Sierra Madre Occidental Mountain range, holds the earliest evidence of popcorn, dating back more than 5,000 years, suggesting that native people were already enjoying it during that time.

Researchers have discovered that individuals in the region now known as Peru consumed popcorn as early as 6,700 years ago. Evidence of this ancient snacking habit, such as old cobs, husks, stalks, and tassels, was recently found at Paredones and Huaca Prieta, two coastal sites that were previously inhabited by prehistoric settlements. A study discussing these findings was published this week in the Proceedings of the National Academy of Sciences. Upon examining the cobs, the researchers concluded that the ancient inhabitants of these Peruvian sites not only popped their corn but also ground it into flour and possibly prepared it in other ways. However, during this early period of maize's history, it was not a significant part of their diet. This situation would change by the 12th century when maize cultivation became crucial to the rise and expansion of the Inca Empire throughout Peru.

While in the South Americas, popcorn and corn held a special place in the lives of the Aztec and Mayan civilizations. The Aztec people used popcorn for various purposes, often as an offering to their gods during religious ceremonies. Aztec priests would even wear elaborate headdresses adorned with popcorn as part of their rituals. In addition to its spiritual significance, popcorn was also enjoyed as a food staple to the point that they even have a word for the popping sound, "totopoca."

The Mayans revered maize, which was the cornerstone of their civilization. They cultivated various types of maize and used these in religious ceremonies, offering it to their deities, and also consumed it as a part of their daily diet. Although there are no specific traces of popcorn use among the Mayans, they held maize in high regard, and their mythology even includes stories about humans being created from maize.

How Popcorn Evolved: From Farming to Technological Innovations

The early settlers of America readily adopted corn, including the popcorn variety, as a staple crop. They learned how to grow and nurture it, ensuring its place in the diets of innumerable people for generations. With the advent of the steel plow in the mid-19th century, which could slice through the most tenacious vegetation, Midwest agriculture experienced a profound transformation. In states like Nebraska, Iowa, and Indiana, corn, especially the kind that could be popped, became a precious cash crop, earning it the nickname "prairie gold." In 1917, this appellation became so deeply entrenched in the region that it inspired a literary work, Prairie Gold, a compilation of poems and stories produced by the Iowa Press and Authors' Club, celebrating the area's abundant corn production.

The traditional method of popping corn in pots over a fire underwent a period of innovation during the 19th century. Frederick J. Myers, a Kentucky resident, patented a corn-popping contraption with a stay-cool handle in 1875. However, popcorn's true popularity would not skyrocket until vendors could easily carry their popping machines with them. In 1885, Charles Cretors from Chicago invented the portable electric machine that used oil to pop kernels, allowing vendors to follow crowds and maximize profits with ease. In 1893, Cretors improved the design by adding a mechanism that buttered and salted the popcorn as it popped.

Several subsequent patents demonstrated the challenges inventors faced in refining the appearance and taste of popcorn. In 1892, James T. Nvoods from Utah filed a patent for a machine that enveloped freshly popped corn in a sugar syrup, which extended the snack's shelf life. The syrupy coating separated the kernels, enabling them to be stored in boxes or packages without becoming damp or dusty. Concurrently, the two brothers explored innovative ways to flavor popcorn. Frederick and Lewis Rueckheim, originally from Germany, sold small quantities of popcorn made using a handheld popper. In 1896, they concocted a winning formula: Cracker Jack, a blend of crispy popcorn and salty peanuts covered in molasses.

The 20th century witnessed a surge of popcorn-related patents, each aiming to improve the product, or the tools used in its creation. Over time, individual vendors and commercial enterprises built on this groundwork, employing technology to cement popcorn's status as a ubiquitous, iconic snack that could be mass-marketed. However, during this period, popcorn vendors primarily relied on street fairs, festivals, and sports events for their revenue. Little did they know that Hollywood would soon revolutionize the course of popcorn's history forever.

The Popcorn and Cinema Connection

The 1920s saw a significant expansion of the movie industry, with approximately 20 thousand movie theaters opening across America. Weekly attendance reached 25 million moviegoers by 1925, presenting a lucrative opportunity for snack vendors who typically set up their stalls at sporting events or festivals. These enterprising vendors began selling their treats outside movie theaters, catching the attention of theater owners.

Initially, many movie theaters had luxuriously carpeted lobbies designed to emulate the grand theater experience. To avoid greasy spills from snacks and drinks, most theaters banned food and beverages outright. However, this prohibition would soon change due to a major shift in the movie industry.

In the late 1920s, sound technology, including dialogue, music, and sound effects, revolutionized cinema. This innovation led to a massive boom in the industry, with weekly moviegoing soaring to 90 million people in 1930, marking the beginning of the Golden Age of cinema. Unfortunately, the shift to sound proved challenging for some smaller or rural theaters, which could not afford the new technology and had to close down. The surviving movie theaters began to cater to a broader audience by shifting their focus from a luxurious atmosphere to a more accessible one, offering popcorn and soda as affordable indulgences.

As the Great Depression took hold, popcorn became a popular "affordable luxury" for millions of Americans, priced at just 10 cents per bag. Struggling to stay afloat, movie theaters eventually relented and began renting portions of their lobbies to popcorn and snack vendors. This decision helped boost their revenues during a challenging economic period.

Stories of wealth acquired through popcorn sales during the Depression emerged with some basis in reality. For example, one farmer managed to buy back his farms with his earnings from popcorn sales. Another story tells of a theater chain that earned $190,000 from popcorn in some locations while its snack-free theaters went bankrupt. One Kansas City vendor secured an impressive annual income (equivalent to nearly $230,000 today) after successfully negotiating with a local theater to sell popcorn to moviegoers.

Over time, theaters began to offer their own refreshments, permanently intertwining concessions, and movie tickets. They even took losses on ticket sales to boost attendance, encouraging patrons to spend money on the more profitable concessions. This practice continues today, with theaters selling popcorn at a markup between 800 and 1,500%, as distributors claim a considerable percentage of ticket sales. As popcorn became a mainstay in movie theater lobbies, its tantalizing aroma became an iconic part of the cinema experience, forever connecting popcorn and movies in the minds of audiences worldwide.

The Birth of the Modern Popcorn Industry

As popcorn evolved from an ancient snack to an American favorite, the industry adapted to meet the demands of a growing market. This section will explore the development of the first popcorn brands, the impact of microwave popcorn on the industry, and the influence of marketing and advertising on popcorn's popularity.

Popcorn at Christmas

We love Christmas around our house and have been known to go over the top with decorations which includes putting up over 20 Christmas trees throughout the house decorated in all different themes.

The tradition of stringing popcorn around a Christmas tree has a charming and nostalgic history that dates back many years. It is believed to have originated in the 19th century when families used simple and natural decorations to adorn their Christmas trees. Popcorn, readily available and affordable, became a popular choice. Families would gather around the fireplace, threading needles with long strands of popcorn and carefully stringing them together. This humble decoration added a touch of rustic beauty to the tree, creating a warm and inviting ambiance in the home. The process of stringing popcorn became a cherished holiday activity, a time for loved ones to come together and bond over a shared task. As time went on, more ornate and elaborate decorations became available, but the tradition of stringing popcorn persevered, serving as a reminder of simpler times and the joy of handmade ornaments. Today, stringing popcorn around the Christmas tree has become a cherished tradition for many, evoking a sense of nostalgia and a connection to the past while also adding a touch of homemade charm to holiday decorations. While we have over 20 Christmas Trees, we haven't gone down the path of decorating them with popcorn yet, but you never know.

The Emergence of the First Popcorn Brands

Between the late 1800s and early 1900s, popcorn made the shift from being a go-to theater snack to a popular treat enjoyed at home. This transition was marked by the founding of several popcorn brands. One of the first commercial popcorn brands was Iowa's Albert Dickinson Co., but they became better known as Big Buster and Little Buster in the 1880s as they started selling under these names. The success of this venture paved the way for other popcorn brands to emerge.

Orville Redenbacher and Charles Bowman introduced their eponymous brand in 1970, which became a household name thanks to its premium-quality kernels and iconic packaging featuring Redenbacher's image. The brand's commitment to using only the finest kernels and innovative farming techniques helped it gain a loyal following and solidify its place in the market.

The Impact of Microwave Popcorn on the Industry

In 1945, Percy Spencer, an engineer at Raytheon, accidentally discovered that microwaves could cook food when a candy bar in his pocket melted while he was working on magnetron tubes. This discovery eventually laid the foundation for microwave ovens, which would go on to revolutionize home cooking and leave a lasting impact on the popcorn industry.

These microwave ovens became more popular in the 1960s to 1970s and brought about a significant change in the lifestyles of people. Popcorn manufacturers begin to seize the opportunity provided by this innovative technology by incorporating it with how they pop popcorn kernels. This was seen in 1981, wherein the first microwave popcorn bags were introduced, giving families an effortless way to enjoy fresh, hot popcorn at home. This allowed them to cook up a tasty treat with minimal effort and time without compromising on quality or flavor.

In 1981, microwave popcorn burst onto the scene, offering consumers a convenient and efficient way to indulge in their favorite snack. The convenience of microwave popcorn led to a spike in demand, and by the mid-1980s, microwaves could be found in more than half of all American homes. This widespread adoption, combined with the simplicity of use and consistent results, propelled microwave popcorn sales to new heights.

Microwave popcorn offered several key advantages over traditional stovetop preparation methods, including faster cooking times, consistent results, and the ability to pop virtually all the kernels in the bag. The pre-packaged, single-use bags also made portion control and clean-up a breeze, further enhancing the appeal of microwave popcorn for busy households.

As microwave popcorn gained popularity, manufacturers began to experiment with various flavors, textures, and additives, such as butter, cheese, and caramel coatings. This expanded range of options allowed consumers to recreate the taste of their favorite cinema or fairground popcorn in the comfort of their own homes.

Companies such as Act II, Orville Redenbacher, and Pop Secret dominated the microwave popcorn market, offering a variety of flavors and package sizes to cater to diverse tastes and preferences. The introduction of microwave popcorn also led to the development of new technologies and packaging materials to ensure even cooking and prevent scorching.

The Influence of Marketing and Advertising on Popcorn's Popularity

Marketing and advertising have played a crucial role in the rise of popcorn's popularity. The early success of brands like Big Buster and Little Buster can be attributed to effective marketing strategies that focused on the quality and taste of their products.

In the 20th century, advertising campaigns helped popcorn brands connect with consumers on a personal level. The use of catchy slogans, memorable jingles, and eye-catching visuals made popcorn an irresistible treat for many. For instance, Orville Redenbacher's marketing campaigns emphasized the brand's dedication to quality by featuring the founder's image on packaging and in commercials, making the brand synonymous with premium popcorn.

With the rise of television and later the internet, advertising campaigns grew more sophisticated, targeting specific demographics and using celebrity endorsements. Pop Secret, for example, partnered with Disney to create limited-edition popcorn tins adorned with beloved characters, appealing to both kids and adults.

Social media has also contributed to popcorn's popularity, with brands using platforms like Facebook, Instagram, and Twitter to connect with consumers, share recipes, and promote new products. Viral challenges, such as the "popcorn trick shot" phenomenon on TikTok, have further boosted popcorn's visibility and appeal.

Popcorn Meets Television

With the widespread adoption of television in the 1950s, families gathered around their living room sets to watch their favorite shows and movies. This new form of home entertainment created a demand for snack foods that could be easily enjoyed while watching TV. Popcorn, with its established link to the movie-going experience, was a natural choice for many households.

TV commercials also played a significant role in promoting popcorn as the perfect snack for home viewing. Advertisements highlighting the ease of popping corn at home and showcasing various brands of popcorn quickly made their way into regular TV programming. With its irresistible aroma and satisfying crunch, popcorn quickly became synonymous with a cozy night in front of the television.

The Digital Age and the Ongoing Evolution of Home Popcorn Consumption

With the rise of the internet and the advent of streaming services, the way people consume media at home has continued to evolve. Binge-watching television shows and streaming movies have become common pastimes, and popcorn has remained a popular accompaniment to these activities.

In response to the changing landscape of home entertainment, popcorn manufacturers and retailers have diversified their offerings to cater to a wide range of tastes and dietary preferences. Organic, non-GMO, and gluten-free popcorn options have emerged to cater to the growing demand for healthier snack alternatives. At the same time, gourmet popcorn brands offer an array of unique and adventurous flavors, such as sriracha, truffle, and even chocolate-covered varieties.

Popcorn subscription services and curated gift boxes have also gained popularity in recent years, giving consumers a convenient way to try new flavors and enjoy their favorite popcorn varieties delivered right to their doorstep. These services have capitalized on popcorn's popularity as a home entertainment snack, offering a fun and engaging way for consumers to explore the ever-expanding world of popcorn.

In conclusion, the history of popcorn's integration into home entertainment showcases its adaptability and lasting appeal. From its early days as a cherished cinema snack to its current status as a versatile and widely enjoyed treat for home viewing, popcorn has proven that it has the staying power to remain a popular choice for entertainment-seekers in various settings. With ongoing innovation in flavors, preparation methods, and delivery options, it's clear that popcorn will continue to be a beloved snack for years to come.

Popcorn Festivities: Celebrating the Love for a Timeless Snack

In this section, we'll explore various celebrations and festivities dedicated to popcorn, a beloved snack that transcends generations. These events showcase the passion and creativity of popcorn enthusiasts as they come together to honor a timeless treat that has brought joy to so many.

The Marion Popcorn Festival: A Fun-Filled Celebration of Popcorn and Community

Every year, Marion, Ohio, hosts the largest popcorn fair in the world, known as the Marion Popcorn Festival. Established in 1981, this cherished event draws thousands of visitors annually to celebrate the rich history and cultural impact of popcorn. Marion is home to the Wyandot Popcorn Museum and has a longstanding tradition of popcorn production. Thus, it is only proper that it hosts the festival.

Marion, affectionately known as the "Popcorn Capital of the World," is proud to host the festival, thanks to its rich popcorn history and the Wyandot Popcorn Museum located there.

Spanning three days in early September, the Marion Popcorn Festival promises a whole lot of fun for folks of all ages. With live music, amusement rides, parades, and fireworks, there's something for everyone to enjoy.

A key attraction at the festival is the parade, featuring an assortment of floats, marching bands, and community groups, all putting their imaginative flair and love for popcorn on display. The parade route winds through downtown Marion, filling the streets with a festive buzz for all to revel in.

Another crowd-pleaser is the Popcorn Cooking Contest, where contestants compete to whip up the most unique and tasty popcorn-based dishes. Showcasing their culinary prowess and creativity, participants use popcorn as the main ingredient of their creations. The competition is intense, and visitors are often amazed by the innovative recipes and tantalizing flavors presented.

The Marion Popcorn Festival not only honors the importance of popcorn in the region but also serves as a testament to the power of community spirit. Through the dedication and hard work of countless volunteers, the festival continues to grow and thrive, providing a cherished annual tradition for residents and visitors alike. With its exciting blend of attractions, entertainment, and of course, popcorn, the Marion Popcorn Festival is a celebration that truly captures the essence of this iconic snack. As visitors gather each year to enjoy the festivities, the festival stands as a reminder of the enduring appeal and cultural significance of popcorn, uniting people from near and far in a shared love for this simple yet delightful treat.

The Valparaiso Popcorn Festival: Honoring a Popcorn Legend

The Valparaiso Popcorn Festival, held annually in Valparaiso, Indiana, is a vibrant celebration that honors the town's connection to Orville Redenbacher, the legendary popcorn entrepreneur who made Valparaiso his home. Orville Redenbacher's dedication to perfecting popcorn and his commitment to high-quality ingredients earned him a place in the hearts of popcorn enthusiasts worldwide. The festival is a lively, family-friendly affair that pays tribute to his legacy and the town's rich popcorn history.

The event typically takes place on the first Saturday after Labor Day in September, drawing in thousands of visitors from across the country. The festivities kick off with the Popcorn Panic, a 5-mile run and a 5K walk that attracts fitness enthusiasts and casual walkers alike. This fun and energetic start to the day sets the tone for the entire festival.

National Popcorn Day: A Toast to America's Favorite Snack

On January 19th each year, popcorn lovers across the United States come together to celebrate National Popcorn Day. This day of popcorn appreciation highlights the versatile and delicious nature of popcorn as people share their favorite recipes, flavors, and popcorn memories on social media. Many popcorn companies also take part in the celebration, offering special deals and promotions to entice customers and generate buzz around their products.

The Growing Popularity of Gourmet Popcorn and Flavored Varieties

Gourmet popcorn is all about lovingly crafting small batches with the finest ingredients and tons of care, bringing a delightful experience to popcorn enthusiasts everywhere. Many brands in this niche are big on using locally sourced, sustainable ingredients while also coming up with imaginative flavor combos that hit the spot for modern, discerning taste buds.

Over the past few years, quite a few gourmet popcorn brands have made a name for themselves and gained fans. Brands such as Garrett Popcorn Shops, Popcornopolis, and Kernels Gourmet Popcorn have become well-known names, with their products being highly sought after by consumers for their distinct flavors and premium ingredients.

Popcorn as a Healthy Snack Option

Popcorn's role in the health and wellness movement is primarily due to its numerous health benefits when compared to other snack options. When prepared without excessive amounts of oil, butter, or salt, popcorn is a low-calorie, high-fiber snack rich in nutrients like vitamins, minerals, and antioxidants. These qualities make popcorn a popular choice among health-conscious consumers seeking nutritious and satisfying snacks.

Air-popped popcorn is particularly healthy, as it contains minimal fat and calories while still providing a satisfying crunch. Many health experts recommend air-popped popcorn as a guilt-free snack option for those watching their weight or looking to increase their fiber intake. In addition to its nutritional benefits, popcorn is naturally gluten-free, making it a suitable snack for those with celiac disease or gluten intolerance.

The health benefits of popcorn have led to the development of various healthy popcorn brands and products. Companies like SkinnyPop and Boom Chicka Pop have built their reputation on providing health-conscious consumers with guilt-free popcorn options that are low in calories, fat, and sodium while still delivering delicious flavors. The success of these brands highlights the growing demand for healthier popcorn options in today's health and wellness-conscious society.

Popping Profits: The Economic Impact of Popcorn Production

As we've seen in previous sections, popcorn has found a special place in the hearts and stomachs of millions. Because of this, it became one of the world's most cherished snacks. However, it is also important to note that beyond its delightful taste and satisfying crunch, popcorn has also played a considerable role in shaping the global economy. In this part, we'll take a closer look at how the simple popcorn kernel has evolved into a booming industry with far-reaching consequences.

The American Popcorn Pioneers

For a long time, the United States has played a major role in the popcorn business, as the majority of the world's popcorn is produced here. With 25 states cultivating the crop, Nebraska leads the way, responsible for 44% of all popcorn production. It generates an impressive 353.7 million pounds of popcorn each year. Other major popcorn-producing states include Indiana, Illinois, Ohio, and Missouri, all contributing to the nation's thriving popcorn industry. The economic impact of popcorn production in these states is considerable, generating job opportunities for farmers, processing plant workers, and various other industry professionals.

The beloved snack even became the official state snack of both Illinois and Indiana, further highlighting its cultural significance. Moreover, Pulaski County in Indiana has been recognized as the Popcorn Capital of America.

International Expansion: Popcorn's Global Reach

While the United States remains a powerful player in the popcorn industry, other countries have also started to embrace this lucrative crop. Argentina, South Africa, and Ukraine are just a few examples of countries that have begun producing and exporting popcorn, tapping into the worldwide demand for this delicious snack. This international expansion has led to increased competition in the popcorn market, sparking innovation in production methods, packaging, and marketing strategies. As a result, consumers around the globe can now enjoy diverse popcorn products and flavors, all while fueling economic growth in countries that produce and export these.

Looking Ahead: The Future of Popcorn Production

As the popcorn industry continues to expand and evolve, so does its economic impact. With the emergence of health-conscious consumers, many popcorn producers capitalize on the demand for healthier snack alternatives.

Technological advancements in farming and processing methods are also expected to shape the future of popcorn production, leading to increased efficiency and sustainability. As the industry continues to adapt and innovate, the economic impact of popcorn production will undoubtedly remain a significant force in the global economy.

Popcorn's Lasting Legacy

From its humble beginnings as a straightforward snack to its present status as a global sensation, popcorn has left an indelible mark on the world's economy.

Popcorn production has truly taken off, with a continuous demand for new and tantalizing flavors fueling a booming industry that supports a multitude of jobs and generates significant revenue.

The economic influence of popcorn stretches way beyond the major US popcorn producers, extending its reach across the globe. As the industry adapts to shifting consumer tastes and technological advancements, popcorn's role in the worldwide economy is set to stay strong.

To sum it up, the tale of popcorn is one of transformation, tenacity, and growth. This humble kernel has captured the hearts and taste buds of millions, all while fostering a lively and economically important industry. Looking ahead, it's evident that popcorn's journey is far from over, and its impact on the global economy will be felt for years to come.

Chapter 3

Fun Facts About Popcorn

Popcorn is a snack that has been enjoyed by people all around the world for centuries. From movie theaters to carnivals, from cozy nights to big gatherings, popcorn has become a versatile and beloved treat. In this chapter, we'll explore some fascinating and fun facts about popcorn that you probably never knew. Despite how simple this snack may look like, there is a lot to know about it so read on.

Useful War Snack

During World War II, Americans consumed three times the usual amount of popcorn due to sugar being sent overseas for U.S. troops, leaving little for candy production.

The Science of Popcorn

Uncover the captivating science behind popcorn, exploring the unique properties and processes that transform a humble kernel into a delightful, fluffy treat.

Explosive Kernels

People used to believe that a small demon lived inside popcorn kernels, causing them to explode when angered. However, these kernels pop because each contains a small amount of water trapped inside its hard shell. When heated, the water turns into steam, creating pressure that causes the kernel to explode and turn inside out.

The Perfect Temperature

The ideal popping temperature for popcorn is around 356°F (180°C). At this temperature, the pressure inside the kernel reaches around

135 psi, leading to a perfect pop. Additionally, for a kernel to pop, its moisture content needs to be between 13.5% and 14%

Varicty matters

Not all corn can be used to make popcorn. There are four primary types of corn: dent, flint, sweet, and popcorn. Popcorn's scientific name is zea mays everta, and it is the only corn variety that will pop.

Size Matters

When popped, popcorn kernels can expand up to 40 times their original size.

Jumping Kernels

Popcorn kernels can pop up to three feet in the air!

Proper Storage

To maintain the ideal moisture content for popping, avoid storing unpopped popcorn kernels in the refrigerator.

Popcorn Shapes

Most popcorn comes in two basic shapes when popped: butterfly (or snowflake) and mushroom. Butterfly popcorn has "wings" and a light crispy texture, while mushroom popcorn is round with a large, rough surface area and can handle a variety of toppings.

Popcorn and the American Culture

Explore the deep-rooted connection between popcorn and American culture, examining the snack's iconic status and its influence on various aspects of society, from cinema to sports events.

The United States is a Popcorn-Loving Nation

Americans consume over 17 billion quarts of popcorn annually, enough to fill the Empire State Building 18 times. To add, in 2020, 67 million Americans consumed six or more bags of popcorn.

Popcorn Goes to The Fair

Popcorn gained popularity in the United States during the 19th century, particularly at fairs and carnivals. Street vendors would sell freshly popped popcorn in bags or boxes.

The Bestselling Popcorn for Americans

Orville Redenbacher is the most popular popcorn brand in the United States, with 63.59 million Americans consuming it in 2020, followed by Pop Secret, with 49.16 million consumers.

Celebrating Popcorns

January 19th is recognized as National Popcorn Day. At the same time, October is designated as National Popping Popcorn Month.

The Nutritional Value of Popcorn

Learn about popcorn's health benefits and nutritional content, highlighting how this wholesome snack can be an excellent addition to a balanced diet when prepared and consumed mindfully.

A Whole Grain Snack

Popcorn is a whole grain, which means it contains all three components of the grain kernel: the bran, the germ, and the endosperm. Whole grains are a good source of fiber and nutrients. Aside from this, it is gluten-free. Gluten-free foods are suitable for individuals with gluten sensitivity or celiac disease, an autoimmune disorder where the ingestion of gluten leads to damage in the small intestine.

Low in Calories

Plain air-popped popcorn is low in calories, with only about 30 calories per cup. This makes it a great alternative to other, more calorie-dense snacks.

Nutrient-Rich

Popcorn contains lots of various vitamins and minerals, such as B vitamins, magnesium, and phosphorus. It also contains antioxidants, particularly polyphenols, which have been linked to various health benefits.

Protein-Packed

To consume a full serving of protein from popcorn, you'll need to eat about three cups of this delectable snack.

Crazy Flavors and Innovations

Discover the wild world of popcorn innovations and flavors, revealing the creative twists and turns that have transformed a simple snack into an exciting, ever-evolving culinary adventure.

DIY Flavor Experimentation

Many popcorn enthusiasts have taken to experimenting with their own flavor combinations at home, using spices, herbs, and other ingredients to create unique and personalized popcorn experiences. Meanwhile, mainstream brands are taking flavor innovation to new heights with their offbeat offerings. Among their most unusual flavors is the notorious Pregnancy Mix popcorn, which features an unexpected blend of ice cream and dill pickle-flavored popcorn.

We prefer to pop different flavors of popcorn and experiment with multiple products and seasonings to make wonderful creations. We get our inspiration from everyday foods, online research, and from friends and family who like to give us different suggestions and ideas.

It's all about experimentation. Sometimes our flavors come out tasting terrible, but that doesn't stop us from trying out the next idea. We just keep poppin'!

Unique Popcorn-Infused Dishes

There are weird but fascinating dishes that emerged as a culinary trend, with innovative chefs and adventurous home cooks experimenting with this versatile ingredient in a range of unique dishes. Examples include fish coated with a popcorn crust for added texture and flavor, hearty popcorn soups or chowders that provide an interesting twist to classic recipes, and delightful popcorn ice cream, where the familiar taste of popcorn complements the creamy dessert for a truly unforgettable treat.

Famous Popcorn Moments

Popcorn has made numerous appearances in films and television shows throughout the years. Memorable moments include the popcorn-filled house in "Real Genius" (1985). In order to execute the scene in the movie, Coolidge, the movie's director, mentioned that the production team had to make popcorn for six weeks during filming to gather enough for the climactic moment. Furthermore, they constructed a house with hydraulic capabilities, allowing popcorn to "explode" from every entrance and window.

World Records and Popcorn Trivia

Dive into the realm of popcorn trivia and world records, celebrating the incredible achievements, fun facts, and astounding stories that surround this universally cherished snack.

Largest Popcorn Ball

Lar Sac City, Iowa, may not be famous for many things, but it takes great pride in one particular attraction - the world's largest popcorn ball. This massive popcorn ball, housed in a shed, attracts visitors from all over, thanks to billboards along nearby highways, and boosts local businesses with tourism revenue.

Estimated to weigh around 9,370 pounds, the popcorn ball has a diameter of eight feet and a circumference exceeding 24 feet. In February 2009, over 250 volunteers spent 12 hours and 40 minutes rebuilding the sculpture, using 900 pounds of popcorn, more than 2,500 pounds of sugar, and 1,400 pounds of syrup.

Un-popped Kernel Nicknames

Un-popped kernels are sometimes referred to as "old maids" or "spinsters."

Popcorn as a Staple in Homes

Popcorn was a popular breakfast food during the late 19th and early 20th centuries, consumed like cereal today.

Unbelievable Guinness World Record

The longest popcorn string measures 1,200 ft. (365.76 m). Speaking of popcorn strings, it would take over 352,028,160 popcorn kernels to create a trail of popcorn from New York City to Los Angeles

Popcorn has proven itself to be more than just a delectable and satisfying snack – it is a fascinating food that boasts an extensive history, intriguing scientific properties, and a powerful cultural impact. With a rich past that stretches back thousands of years, popcorn has played a starring role in the development of global cuisine, entertainment, and even art. As you enjoy your next bowl of popcorn, remember to savor not only the enticing flavors and textures but also the awe-inspiring journey that each kernel has taken to reach your taste buds. This remarkable snack truly transcends time and space, uniting people across generations and continents in a shared love for this unique, versatile, and utterly delightful treat.

Chapter 4

Popcorn Games

Popcorn isn't just a delicious snack; it's also the key ingredient to some seriously fun and creative games. Whether you're looking for ways to liven up a movie night, host a popcorn-themed party, or simply enjoy some quality time with friends and family, these popcorn-inspired games are sure to pop your boredom away!

Popcorn Toss

Let's start with a classic: Popcorn Toss! This game is a delightful combination of skill and luck. Set up a target, whether it's a bucket, a hoop, or even a large mixing bowl, and take turns trying to toss popcorn kernels into it.

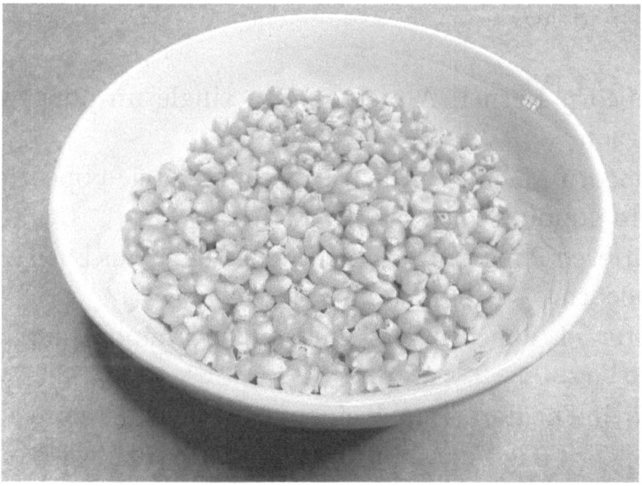

Assign different point values to different distances for added excitement. It's a game that anyone can enjoy, regardless of age.

Popcorn Relay Race

Get your heart racing with a Popcorn Relay Race. Divide your group into teams and give each team a spoon and a container filled with popcorn kernels. The challenge? Players must transfer popcorn from one container to another using only the spoon, without dropping a single kernel. The first team to successfully transfer all their popcorn wins!

Popcorn Bingo

Popcorn Bingo is perfect for a relaxed evening with friends or family. Create bingo cards with popcorn-related images or facts, like a popcorn kernel, a popcorn machine, or a bag of popcorn. Call out descriptions, and players mark their cards accordingly. The first person to get five in a row yells "Bingo!" and wins a popcorn-themed prize.

Bingo image ideas:

- Popcorn Kernel: A picture of a single un-popped popcorn kernel.
- Popcorn Machine: Illustration of a classic popcorn machine with popping corn.
- Buttered Popcorn: A depiction of a delicious bowl of buttered popcorn.
- Caramel Popcorn: An image of caramel-coated popcorn clusters.
- Movie Theater: A small cinema or movie theater icon.
- Popcorn Bag: A graphic of a paper bag filled with popcorn.
- Popcorn Bucket: A picture of a colorful popcorn bucket with kernels.
- Popcorn Box: An illustration of a box of popcorn often found at movie theaters.
- Popcorn Cart: A classic popcorn cart with a popcorn vendor.

Popcorn Pictionary

Combine your love for art and popcorn with Popcorn Pictionary. This twist on the classic drawing game has players drawing popcorn-themed words or phrases while their teammates guess what's being illustrated. Get ready for some hilarious interpretations and lots of laughter.

Popcorn Memory Game

Test your memory skills with the Popcorn Memory Game. Create pairs of cards with images or names of different popcorn flavors or popcorn-related items. Place them face down and take turns flipping two cards over. If you find a match, you get to keep the pair. The player with the most pairs at the end wins.

Popcorn Trivia Quiz

Think you know everything there is to know about popcorn? Put your knowledge to the test with a Popcorn Trivia Quiz. Prepare a list of questions about popcorn's history, types, and cultural significance. You can make it a competitive game with prizes for the winners or a fun learning experience for all.

Popcorn Sculpture Contest

Let your creativity run wild with a Popcorn Sculpture Contest. Provide your participants with a pile of popped popcorn and various art supplies like glue, markers, and colored paper. Challenge them to create sculptures or artwork using popcorn as the main component. You'll be amazed at the imaginative creations that emerge.

Popcorn Tasting Challenge

Elevate your popcorn game with a Popcorn Tasting Challenge. Blindfold participants and offer them a variety of popcorn flavors, from classic buttered to exotic gourmet options. Challenge them to guess the ingredients or seasonings used in each one. It's a delicious way to explore new flavors and have a taste bud adventure.

These popcorn-inspired games and activities are perfect for adding a dose of fun and creativity to your gatherings or solo popcorn adventures. So, grab a bowl of your favorite popcorn and let the games begin!

Chapter 5

Popcorn in POPular Culture

Popcorn has become synonymous with entertainment, whether it's a night at the movies, binge-watching television, or listening to music at a festival. This iconic snack has weaved its way into popular culture, becoming a symbol of leisure and togetherness. Let's explore the origins of popcorn's popularity, its role in various entertainment settings, and how it has inspired the creative arts, making its mark on film, television, and music.

Short Fascinating History of How Popcorn Became a Staple in Movies

Today, concession sales, particularly popcorn, are vital to theaters' financial success. While ticket sales are shared with studios, the profits from snacks are what keep theaters afloat. This is why concession prices are often steep, as they are a primary source of income for theaters.

The rise of home video brought new challenges for Hollywood and the theater industry, with fears that people would watch movies at home instead of in theaters. However, the allure of the theater experience persisted, and popcorn became an integral part of movie nights at home. Whether it's stovetop or microwave popcorn, people continue to crave the sensory satisfaction of enjoying popcorn while watching a film.

The connection between popcorn and movies is a fascinating tale of persistence, innovation, and cultural evolution. As the movie industry continues to adapt to new technologies and consumer preferences, one thing is certain: the irresistible combination of popcorn and movies is here to stay.

Popcorn and the Silver Screen

Since the early days of cinema, popcorn has been a staple of the moviegoing experience. The smell of freshly popped corn wafts through the air, tempting us with its buttery aroma. Iconic films have paid homage to popcorn, either through memorable scenes or by featuring it prominently in their marketing materials.

Popcorn has become a symbol of watching movies, as audiences eagerly munch on their popcorn while being thrilled and engaged by the action on screen. The 1996 film, Scream perfectly captures this sentiment during the conversation of the character, Casey, with an anonymous caller on her phone. This was their conversation, 'Caller: You're making popcorn? Casey: Uh huh. Caller: I only eat popcorn at the movies. Casey: Well, I'm getting ready to watch a video." Even when Casey was simply watching a short video rather than a full-length movie, popcorn remained a go-to snack to enjoy alongside any form of moving images.

Popcorn in Television

Popcorn's ubiquity in popular culture extends beyond the silver screen and into the realm of television. From sitcoms to dramas, our favorite characters often share their most memorable moments with a bowl of popcorn in hand.

The beloved television series Gilmore Girls frequently featured the mother-daughter duo of Lorelai and Rory bonding as they watched their favorite films and television shows. A massive bowl of popcorn was one of their snacks here. Not only does it show that popcorn is indeed a movie night snack, but it also goes to show how the two are relatable, as we would all go for popcorn when watching a movie.

In the realm of reality television, the iconic show Survivor has also found a way to incorporate popcorn into its rich tapestry of challenges, alliances, and dramatic moments. Throughout its long run, the show has captivated audiences with its unique blend of physical and mental competitions, strategic gameplay, and unforgettable characters. Amidst all the excitement, popcorn has played a subtle yet noteworthy role in the Survivor experience. On one occasion, the show had a survivor cinema wherein the contestants could enjoy a movie with a mountain of popcorn available. This gave birth to an iconic moment in the show where a contestant shoves his face into the popcorn while enjoying the snack. Indeed, who wouldn't do the same when popcorn is in front of you?

Popcorn and Music: From Concerts to Songs

Popcorn's influence on popular culture doesn't stop at film and television; it has also made its mark on the music industry. Outdoor music festivals and concerts often feature popcorn stands, providing fans with a delicious snack as they enjoy their favorite bands.

Lyrics referencing popcorn can be found in various genres, from rap and hip-hop to pop and country. For instance, the 2008 hit "Popcorn" by the Crazy Frog sampled Gershon Kingsley's 1969 instrumental "Popcorn," turning it into a catchy dance tune that achieved worldwide success.

Popcorn's Impact on Fashion and Art

Popcorn's influence on popular culture goes beyond entertainment, making its way into fashion and art. Designers have been inspired by the snack's unique texture and visual appeal, incorporating popcorn-like elements into clothing and accessories. In 2015, fashion label Moschino released a popcorn-themed cape, which quickly became a statement piece for fashion-forward individuals.

Street artists and painters have also embraced popcorn as a subject in their work, often using it as a symbol of Americana or a representation of the entertainment industry. For instance, Burton Morris, is an American artist known for his stylized depictions of popcorn, which can be found in galleries and on the walls of prominent Hollywood establishments.

The captivating history of popcorn and its deep-rooted connection with cinema represents an incredible tale of adaptation, consumer demand, and cultural impact. As the movie industry continues to evolve, facing challenges from emerging technologies, streaming services, and shifting consumer preferences, the timeless pairing of popcorn and movies remains steadfast and cherished.

The relationship between popcorn and movies has not only endured but thrived over time, thanks to the snack's affordability, simplicity, and universal appeal. As popcorn became an integral part of the cinematic experience, it has also become a symbol of shared memories, family outings, and the sheer joy of immersing oneself in the world of film. It is this emotional connection that has helped cement popcorn's status as the quintessential movie snack, both in theaters and at home.

As technology continues to reshape the landscape of entertainment, popcorn has proven its ability to adapt and maintain relevance. With the rise of home entertainment and streaming platforms, popcorn has successfully made the transition from theaters to living rooms around the world. Families and friends now gather to enjoy movie nights, binge-watch their favorite series, or indulge in reality TV marathons, all while sharing a warm, buttery bowl of popcorn.

Moreover, the enduring love for popcorn extends beyond just movies and television. The ubiquity of popcorn at sports events, amusement parks, and various entertainment venues speaks to its adaptability and widespread appeal. Popcorn has become emblematic of numerous shared experiences and happy moments that we cherish in our lives.

As we anticipate the future of cinema and entertainment, it's clear that popcorn will maintain its central role in our collective enjoyment. The unassuming yet potent connection between popcorn and movies celebrates the human bonds we forge, serves as a reminder of life's simple pleasures, and acts as a bridge uniting generations and cultures. This inherent connection ensures that the enchanting partnership of popcorn and movies will continue to thrive, undeterred by any obstacles or transformations the entertainment industry may face.

Chapter 6

Is Popcorn Healthy?

Despite its popularity, many people still have misconceptions about popcorn's nutritional value, often regarding it as a "junk food" or an unhealthy indulgence.

Contrary to these widespread beliefs, popcorn actually offers numerous health benefits when prepared and consumed in moderation. In fact, it's a whole grain packed with essential nutrients, making it a surprisingly healthful snack option. Of course, not all popcorn is created equal; the nutritional value can vary significantly depending on the method of preparation and the toppings used. But when enjoyed mindfully, popcorn can be a guilt-free, nutritious treat.

In this chapter, we'll delve into the surprising health benefits of popcorn, debunking common misconceptions, and exploring why this popular snack is good for you. From its impressive nutrient profile to its potential impact on weight management, heart health, and more, we'll reveal the fascinating truth behind this seemingly humble snack. So grab a bowl of popcorn, sit back, and get ready to discover why popcorn is more than just a tasty treat—it's a snack worth celebrating for its health benefits too.

Health Benefits of Popcorn

Improved Digestion

Popcorn, being a whole grain, retains all three parts of the kernel: the bran, germ, and endosperm. The bran, the outer layer of the kernel, is rich in dietary fiber. Fiber is crucial for a healthy digestive system as it adds bulk to stools and helps food pass smoothly through the digestive tract. Consuming whole grains like popcorn can significantly improve digestion and prevent issues such as constipation, bloating, and irregular bowel movements.

Reducing the Risk of Heart Disease

Popcorn, as a whole grain, offers a range of heart-healthy benefits, thanks to its abundance of nutrients such as fiber, vitamins, and minerals. These nutrients play a role in enhancing cardiovascular health. Studies suggest that individuals who consistently eat whole grains often have a reduced risk of heart disease, partly due to their cholesterol-lowering and blood pressure-reducing effects. By incorporating popcorn into your diet, you can boost your heart health and potentially lower your risk of cardiovascular diseases.

Aiding in Weight Management

With its high fiber and complex carbohydrate content, popcorn can be a helpful ally in managing your weight. Foods rich in fiber promote a sense of fullness, making it less likely that you'll overeat. Additionally, complex carbohydrates are digested more slowly, providing a sustained energy source, and preventing abrupt blood sugar spikes. This satisfying combination of fiber and complex carbs keeps you feeling full for longer periods, making it easier to resist unhealthy snacks and maintain a healthy weight. Aside from this popcorn is a relatively low-calorie snack, especially compared to other popular snack options like chips or candy. Thus, if it is prepared without excessive amounts of oil, butter, or other high-calorie toppings, popcorn can be an excellent choice for those trying to lose weight.

Assists in Blood Sugar Regulation

Popcorn's fiber content can also aid in regulating blood sugar levels by slowing down glucose absorption into the bloodstream. This process helps prevent abrupt spikes in blood sugar and can be especially helpful for individuals with diabetes or those at risk of developing the condition. By incorporating popcorn into your diet, you can savor a delicious snack while also promoting healthy blood sugar control.

Protection Against Free Radicals

Popcorn is a surprisingly rich source of antioxidants, specifically polyphenols. Antioxidants are crucial in combating free radicals, which can cause cellular damage and contribute to the development of chronic diseases like cancer, heart disease, and diabetes. The antioxidants in popcorn can help neutralize these harmful free radicals, supporting overall health and well-being.

Potential Cancer-Fighting Properties

While more research is needed, some studies suggest that the antioxidants in popcorn may have cancer-fighting properties. The polyphenols found in popcorn have been shown to inhibit the growth of cancer cells in laboratory settings. Although more research is required to fully understand the relationship between popcorn and cancer prevention, incorporating antioxidant-rich foods like popcorn into your diet could potentially contribute to a reduced risk of developing certain types of cancer.

Notable Nutrients That Can be Found in Popcorn

Vitamin B complex for energy production.

Popcorn contains several B vitamins, including thiamin, niacin, and folate. These vitamins play a crucial role in energy production by helping your body convert carbohydrates into usable energy. By consuming popcorn, you can support your body's energy production and overall vitality.

Magnesium for nerve and muscle function.

Magnesium is an essential mineral that supports nerve and muscle function, among other vital roles in the body. Popcorn is a good source of magnesium, which means that enjoying this snack can contribute to maintaining healthy nerve and muscle function. Adequate magnesium intake is also associated with improved sleep, reduced muscle cramps, and better bone health.

Iron for blood cell production.

Popcorn contains a small but significant amount of iron, an essential mineral required for blood cell production and the transport of oxygen throughout the body. Consuming iron-rich foods like popcorn can help prevent iron-deficiency anemia and support overall health, particularly for those at risk of iron deficiency, such as pregnant women, vegans, and vegetarians.

How to Enjoy Popcorn in a Healthy Way

Portion Control

Despite popcorn's numerous health benefits, it is essential to practice portion control to ensure you're not consuming too many calories or overindulging in unhealthy toppings. A standard serving size of air-popped popcorn is about 3 cups, which provides around 90-120 calories, depending on the toppings used. By adhering to appropriate portion sizes, you can enjoy popcorn's benefits without jeopardizing your weight management or overall health goals.

Healthy Toppings and Flavorings

Creating a tasty and nutritious popcorn snack is all about selecting the perfect toppings and seasonings. Here are a few ideas to enhance your popcorn while maintaining its healthiness:

Herbs and Spices

Incorporating herbs and spices into your popcorn not only boosts its flavor but also offers added health benefits. Somc popular choices include garlic powder, onion powder, smoked paprika, cumin, turmeric, and black pepper. Fresh herbs like rosemary, thyme, and oregano can also impart a burst of flavor to your popcorn without contributing extra calories or sodium.

Nutritional Yeast

Nutritional yeast boasts a savory, cheese-like flavor, making it a fantastic addition to dishes. Rich in B vitamins and protein, it makes for a nutritious and scrumptious topping for popcorn. To enjoy this guilt-free snack, simply sprinkle a tablespoon or two of nutritional yeast over your air-popped popcorn.

Olive Oil

While air-popped popcorn is the healthiest option, if you prefer oil-popped popcorn, opt for healthier oil options like olive oil. Olive oil is rich in monounsaturated fats, which are considered heart-healthy and can help reduce the risk of cardiovascular disease. Drizzle a small amount of olive oil over your popcorn to add flavor while keeping it nutritious.

Avoiding Unhealthy Additives

To fully enjoy the health benefits of popcorn, it's essential to avoid unhealthy additives that can negate its nutritional value. Here are some additives to steer clear of:

Excessive Salt

Although a small amount of salt can enhance popcorn's flavor, consuming too much sodium can lead to health issues like high blood pressure and heart disease. To keep your popcorn healthy, use minimal salt or opt for salt-free seasonings like herbs and spices.

Artificial Flavors and Colors

Commercially prepared popcorn may contain artificial flavors and colors that offer no nutritional value and can be harmful to your health. When enjoying popcorn, it's best to stick to natural flavorings like herbs, spices, and nutritional yeast to ensure you're reaping its full benefits.

Trans Fats

Trans fats, often found in commercially prepared popcorn and microwave popcorn, can raise LDL ("bad") cholesterol levels and increase the risk of heart disease. To keep your popcorn healthy, avoid products containing trans fats, and choose air-popped popcorn or popcorn made with healthier oils like olive oil.

By following these guidelines, you can enjoy popcorn in a healthy way that allows you to take full advantage of its numerous benefits. Experiment with different combinations of herbs, spices, and other nutritious toppings to create a delicious, satisfying snack that supports your health.

Potential Concerns

While popcorn has numerous health benefits, there are some potential concerns that you should be aware of when incorporating it into your diet.

Dental Issues

Chipped Teeth

Popcorn can occasionally pose dental risks, such as chipped teeth, particularly when consuming partially popped kernels or "old maids." These hard kernels can be surprisingly tough and may cause damage to teeth if bitten into with force. To minimize this risk, be cautious when eating popcorn and avoid biting down on hard kernels.

Popcorn Kernels Stuck in Gums

Another dental concern related to popcorn consumption is the possibility of kernels becoming lodged in your gums or between your teeth. This can cause discomfort, inflammation, and even infection if not promptly addressed. To prevent this issue, be sure to floss and brush your teeth after eating popcorn to dislodge any trapped kernels.

Popcorn-Related Allergies

Although rare, some individuals may have an allergy to corn or corn products, including popcorn. Symptoms of a corn allergy can range from mild, such as itching or hives, to severe, including difficulty breathing or anaphylaxis. If you suspect that you have a corn allergy, consult with an allergist or healthcare professional for proper diagnosis and guidance on managing your allergy.

High Sodium Content in Commercially Prepared Popcorn

Commercially prepared popcorn, particularly pre-packaged and microwave varieties, often contains excessive amounts of sodium. High sodium intake has been linked to increased blood pressure and a higher risk of heart disease. When choosing popcorn, opt for air-popped or homemade versions with minimal salt to avoid excessive sodium consumption. If you prefer commercially prepared popcorn, look for low-sodium options and be mindful of portion sizes.

By incorporating popcorn into your diet as a nutritious snack option, you can enjoy its numerous health benefits without sacrificing taste or satisfaction. Experiment with different healthy toppings and flavor combinations to create a delicious, wholesome treat that supports your overall health and well-being. So, the next time you're looking for a snack, consider reaching for a bowl of popcorn and indulge in its delightful crunch and nourishing benefits.

Chapter 7

Popcorn Flavors

Popcorn, a beloved snack enjoyed around the globe, boasts a remarkable array of flavors and preparation techniques. This timeless treat transcends cultures, unifying people through their love for its delightful crunch and taste. With countless variations in preparation and consumption, popcorn continues to evolve and surprise our taste buds.

Popping Techniques: The Perfect Crunch

The first step to creating irresistible popcorn is mastering the popping method. Different regions around the world have adopted unique techniques to achieve that perfect crunch. For example, air-popped popcorn is popular in the United States for its low-fat appeal, while street vendors in Brazil (known as Pipoqueiros) rely on large, covered pans to create a show-stopping snack. Each method adds a distinct touch to the final product, making the popcorn experience even more enjoyable.

Flavors Galore: The Spice of Life

Once the kernels have been popped to perfection, it's time to add a touch of flavor. From sweet to savory and everything in between, the diverse range of seasonings and toppings is a testament to the world's creativity. In India, masala popcorn is a hit, combining the bold flavors of traditional Indian spices. Over in Japan, a dusting of furikake (a savory Japanese seasoning) transforms popcorn into a uniquely satisfying treat. Even the classic American caramel corn has seen countless variations, such as the indulgent Chicago-style mix combining caramel and cheese popcorn.

Serving It Up: Creative Presentations

Popcorn's versatility extends beyond just flavor, as it can be served in various forms to suit different occasions. The United States boasts a Halloween tradition of making popcorn balls, a festive treat made by binding popcorn together with a sweet syrup. In Colombia, arepas, a type of cornbread, can be stuffed with popcorn for a delicious and unexpected twist.

As we explore the different ways popcorn is flavored, popped, and consumed around the world, it's easy to understand why this humble snack remains universally adored. Its adaptability and endless possibilities continue to captivate food lovers everywhere, ensuring popcorn's place as a global favorite.

Canada

Canada shares many popcorn preferences with its southern neighbor, the United States. Canadian popcorn lovers also enjoy air-popped, microwave, and movie theater popcorn, as well as caramel corn and other flavored varieties. However, Canada has its own unique twist on this classic snack.

Maple syrup flavored popcorn

In true Canadian fashion, maple syrup-flavored popcorn is a popular choice among snackers. This variety features popcorn coated in a deliciously sweet and sticky maple glaze, often with the addition of nuts like pecans or walnuts. Indeed, this flavor pays homage to the country's iconic syrup.

Mexico

Lime and chili-infused Mexican popcorn

Mexico puts its own spin on the classic popcorn snack by incorporating traditional ingredients. This variation is often seasoned with a tangy mix of lime and chili powder, resulting in a zesty and spicy delight. For those craving a snack with a little kick, this flavor-packed combination is a perfect choice.

South America

South America boasts a wealth of culture and culinary diversity, and this is reflected in the region's popcorn creations as well. From the bustling streets of Brazil to the flavorful traditions of Argentina, popcorn in South America is a delightful exploration of flavors and regional specialties.

Brazil

Pipoca - Street vendors

Pipoca, or popcorn in Portuguese, is a popular snack enjoyed by many Brazilians. Street vendors, known as pipoqueiros, can be found on busy streets and public spaces, serving up freshly popped popcorn from their distinctive carts. These carts often feature a large, covered pan where the popcorn is popped using oil, and the pipoqueiro expertly seasons the snack with salt, sugar, or a combination of both.

Sweet popcorn - Pipoca de isopor

Pipoca de isopor, or styrofoam popcorn, is a Brazilian sweet popcorn variety that is known for its light and airy texture reminiscent of styrofoam. This type of popcorn is made by coating the freshly popped kernels in a sugary syrup, creating a sweet and crunchy treat. This unique texture has made pipoca de isopor a favorite among children and adults alike.

Peru

Canchita - Traditional Peruvian popcorn

Canchita is a traditional Peruvian popcorn snack that is made from a special corn variety called maíz chulpe. It's a must try since, unlike regular popcorn, these kernels don't burst when heated. Instead, they puff up and become crunchy. Often seasoned with salt, canchita is a popular complimentary snack in bars, restaurants, and at social events around the country.

Ceviche-inspired popcorn

Many have experimented with popcorn flavors, and many will be shocked when they know that there is popcorn inspired by Peru's famous ceviche. It is a dish that is part of the country's well-loved cuisine and features raw fish marinated in citrus juice and spices. Ceviche-inspired popcorn blends the much-loved snack with flavorful seasonings like lime, chili, cilantro, and onion, crafting a zesty and invigorating delight. This taste sensation celebrates Peru's culinary richness and brings a burst of the country's vibrant cuisine to your palate.

Argentina

Chimichurri popcorn

Argentina's famous chimichurri sauce, a green blend of parsley, garlic, vinegar, and oil, is commonly served with grilled meats. Because of its tasty and savory flavor, combining it with popcorn creates a must–try treat. Though it is uncommon to combine sauces with popcorn, it is perfect for those who want a vegan way to enjoy the sauce without eating meat.

Dulce de leche popcorn

Dulce de leche, a rich and velvety caramel-like sauce, holds a special place in the hearts of Argentinians. When this luscious sauce meets popcorn, it creates a heavenly treat that marries the sweetness of dulce de leche with the light, crispy texture of popcorn. This scrumptious snack is perfect for satisfying the cravings of anyone with a sweet tooth.

Colombia

Mazorca desgranada - Corn-based Street food

While not exactly popcorn, mazorca desgranada is a beloved Colombian street food made from corn. This dish features a base of boiled and seasoned corn kernels topped with various ingredients like cheese, potato sticks, and meat, creating a flavorful and satisfying snack that demonstrates corn's versatility in Colombian cuisine.

Popcorn-filled Arepa de Huevo

Arepas, a type of cornbread, is a staple in Colombian and Venezuelan cuisine. Typically made from cornmeal, inventive cooks have experimented with using popcorn as a base for this popular dish. By grinding popped popcorn into a fine flour and mixing it with other ingredients like eggs and cheese, a popcorn-based arepa de huevo emerges. This creative take on a classic dish, highlights both the adaptability of popcorn and the ingenuity of South American cuisine.

In conclusion, South America offers a delightful assortment of popcorn flavors and traditions that celebrate the continent's rich culinary heritage. From Brazil's iconic street vendors to Colombia's innovative adaptations of traditional dishes, South American popcorn provides a colorful and flavorful sensory journey. These unique and tasty popcorn varieties pay tribute to the continent's love for this versatile snack and showcase the endless possibilities popcorn offers.

Asia

Asia's diverse culinary landscape boasts a wide range of flavors, techniques, and ingredients that have been adapted and integrated into popcorn offerings across the continent. From the bold spices of India to the subtle flavors of Japan, Asia's vibrant culinary landscape showcases an array of flavors, techniques, and ingredients, which have been creatively adapted into popcorn varieties across the continent.

China

Five-Spice Popcorn

With a rich culinary history steeped in flavors and spices, China has much to offer. Five-spice powder, a harmonious blend of star anise, cloves, cinnamon, Sichuan pepper, and fennel seeds, is a staple in Chinese cuisine. Seasoning popcorn with this fragrant and flavorful spice mixture results in a delectable and aromatic snack that represents China's culinary roots. This distinctive popcorn variety is perfect for those eager to delve into the bold and intricate flavors of Chinese cuisine.

Chiu Chow Chili Oil Popcorn

Hailing from the Chiu Chow region of China, Chiu Chow chili oil is a spicy and flavorful condiment revered for its rich, garlicky, and umami-laden taste. Infusing popcorn with Chiu Chow chili oil creates a fiery and savory treat that showcases China's love for bold flavors. This popcorn offers a glimpse into the robust and savory flavors that define Chiu Chow cuisine, paying tribute to China's diverse culinary landscape.

India

Masala popcorn

India's vibrant culinary heritage is renowned for its dynamic and bold spices. Masala popcorn highlights this by using a mix of Indian spices like cumin, coriander, turmeric, and chili powder. The outcome is a spicy, fragrant, and tasty treat that embodies the spirit of Indian cuisine.

Tandoori Popcorn

Drawing inspiration from the traditional Indian tandoor oven cooking method, tandoori popcorn combines the smoky and spicy flavors typically associated with tandoori dishes. This unique popcorn variation offers a taste of India's beloved grilled cuisine in a fun and crunchy snack form.

Jaggery popcorn

Jaggery, an unrefined sugar made from sugarcane, is a frequent ingredient in Indian sweets. Coating popcorn with a jaggery syrup creates a delicious and distinctively sweet snack. This caramel-like treat showcases India's love for rich, indulgent flavors and is perfect for those with a sweet tooth.

Japan

Furikake popcorn

Furikake is a Japanese seasoning blend consisting of a mix of dried fish or other protein, sesame seeds, dried seaweed flakes, sugar and soy sauce.

By sprinkling furikake over popcorn, Japan has created a savory, umami-rich snack that highlights the delicate flavors of Japanese cuisine. This innovative popcorn variety is perfect for those looking to experience the unique flavors of Japan.

Matcha popcorn

Matcha, a finely ground green tea powder, is a staple in Japanese cuisine and is revered for its health benefits and distinct flavor. By dusting popcorn with matcha powder, Japan has created a subtly sweet and earthy snack that is both delicious and uniquely Japanese.

Teriyaki popcorn

Teriyaki, a popular Japanese cooking technique, involves glazing food with a sweet and savory sauce made from soy sauce, mirin, and sugar. Teriyaki popcorn captures the essence of this beloved flavor by coating popcorn in a teriyaki glaze, resulting in a snack that is both sweet and savory.

Japan's Popcorn Craze: Collectible and Creative Popcorn Buckets at Tokyo Disneyland

In Japan, the love for popcorn goes beyond just the flavors. Tokyo Disneyland has played a significant role in igniting the craze for collectible and creative popcorn buckets. Disney-themed popcorn buckets have become hot commodities for visitors at Tokyo Disneyland and other theme parks. Adorned with beloved characters and motifs, these unique containers are cherished by both locals and tourists as treasured souvenirs and collectibles.

These parks offer not just a wide array of popcorn flavors but also the chance to grab limited-edition popcorn buckets. This craze extends beyond the theme parks and has played a role in elevating popcorn's status in Japan as a fun, interactive snack. The popcorn phenomenon showcases the snack's incredible adaptability and ability to bring people together through shared interests, further cementing its place in the hearts of popcorn enthusiasts everywhere.

Korea

Kimchi-flavored popcorn

Kimchi, the well-known fermented vegetable dish, is a cornerstone of Korean cuisine, famous for its bold and tangy taste. Kimchi-flavored popcorn honors this iconic dish by fusing kimchi's flavors with the satisfying crunch of popcorn. This creative snack showcases Korea's passion for bold, spicy flavors and is perfect for those craving a taste of Korean cuisine.

Honey Butter Popcorn

Honey butter chips have taken Korea by storm with their mouthwatering blend of sweet and savory flavors. Applying this irresistible taste to popcorn, Korea has given birth to honey butter popcorn—a scrumptious and addictive snack that's distinctively Korean. This sweet and savory treat is perfect for those who appreciate the harmonious balance of flavors that Korean cuisine has to offer.

Thailand

Thai curry popcorn

Thai cuisine is known for its bold and fragrant flavors, and Thai curry popcorn is no exception. By seasoning popcorn with a blend of Thai curry spices such as lemongrass, galangal, kaffir lime leaves, and chili, this unique popcorn variety captures the essence of Thai cuisine. The harmonious balance of spicy, sweet, and sour flavors in Thai curry popcorn is a delicious tribute to Thailand's rich culinary heritage.

Coconut and curry popcorn

Thai cuisine is celebrated for its rich and flavorful dishes, with coconut and curry as two indispensable ingredients. By combining these flavors with popcorn, a unique snack has been created that showcases Thailand's passion for lively and zesty tastes. The blend of coconut's sweet, creamy notes with the warm, aromatic touch of curry results in a remarkable Thai popcorn experience that's sure to please your taste buds.

The diverse Asian culinary scene has given rise to an incredible variety of popcorn flavors, each reflecting the distinct ingredients and traditions of their respective countries.

From the fiery spices of India to the subtle, refined notes of Japan, these popcorn variations serve as a delicious reminder of Asia's passion for food and culinary innovation. Popcorn enthusiasts worldwide can rejoice in this celebration of Asia's love for the humble snack, as each tasty morsel offers a glimpse into the rich tapestry of flavors that define the region.

Africa

Africa's rich culinary heritage offers a diverse array of flavors, techniques, and ingredients that have been adapted and incorporated into popcorn varieties across the continent. From the spicy and bold flavors of Nigeria to the fragrant and aromatic spices of Morocco, Africa's popcorn varieties showcase the unique flavors and culinary traditions of each country.

Nigeria

Suya-spiced popcorn

Suya, a popular Nigerian street food, consists of skewered, grilled meat seasoned with a spicy and flavorful blend of spices, peanuts, and other ingredients. The flavor brought about by this mixture of seasoning has inspired many to try seasoning popcorn with it. Thus, you can get a glimpse into Nigerian culinary flavors with this simple snack. Also, this distinctive popcorn variety is perfect for those seeking to explore the bold and complex flavors of Nigerian cuisine.

Groundnut popcorn

Groundnuts, or peanuts, are a staple ingredient in Nigerian cuisine and are used to make a variety of dishes, including soups, stews, and snacks. By mixing spicy groundnuts, it creates a unique treat that highlights the country's love for both sweet and savory flavors. The harmony of the crunchy popcorn and the rich, nutty groundnut is a delightful nod to Nigeria's culinary traditions.

South Africa

Biltong-Spiced Popcorn

For those craving a truly unique flavor, biltong-spiced popcorn is the answer. Inspired by biltong, a cherished South African snack made from cured and dried meat, this popcorn variety combines rich and savory flavors. Seasoning popcorn with biltong spices like coriander, black pepper, and vinegar creates a scrumptious and distinctive snack that embodies the essence of biltong. Some even go the extra mile by adding meat fat and peanut brittle for an additional burst of flavor.

Sweet and Spicy Chutney Popcorn

Sweet and spicy chutneys play a central role in South African cuisine, often served as a condiment with various dishes. Simba, a popular South African snack brand, has embraced this flavor profile by crafting sweet and spicy chutney-flavored popcorn.

Morocco

Popcorn with Ras El Hanout

Ras el hanout, translating to "top of the shop" in Arabic, represents a mix of the most exquisite spices from Morocco. Popcorn sprinkled with ras el hanout embodies these vibrant flavors, crafting a one-of-a-kind and mouthwatering snack that highlights Morocco's rich culinary heritage. It's a perfect pick for anyone eager to delve into the unique and intricate flavors that Moroccan cuisine has to offer.

Popcorn with Harissa and Honey

Harissa, a spicy and flavorful chili paste, plays a significant role in Moroccan cuisine and is frequently used to add heat and depth to a variety of dishes. When paired with honey, harissa lends itself to a sweet and spicy popcorn delight that harmoniously balances the chili paste's heat with the honey's natural sweetness. This delightful snack showcases Morocco's passion for bold and lively flavors and is sure to entice the taste buds of popcorn enthusiasts around the world.

Africa's diverse culinary landscape has given rise to a wide array of unique and delicious popcorn flavors. Each country's distinct ingredients and culinary traditions are showcased in their popcorn offerings, providing snackers with a taste of Africa's rich culinary history. From the bold and spicy flavors of Nigeria to the fragrant and aromatic spices of Morocco

Oceania

Oceania, encompassing Australia, New Zealand, and the Pacific Islands, boasts a vibrant and diverse culinary scene. Drawing inspiration from the region's unique ingredients and cultural influences, Oceania has given rise to a variety of popcorn flavors that reflect the distinct character of each country. From Australia's iconic

Vegemite to New Zealand's beloved hokey pokey, these popcorn creations celebrate the rich culinary traditions of Oceania.

Australia

Vegemite Popcorn

Vegemite, the savory, yeast extract-based spread that's an Aussie favorite, has inspired the creation of Vegemite popcorn. This intriguing blend combines the distinct umami taste of Vegemite with the crunchy satisfaction of popcorn, resulting in a savory snack that pays tribute to Australia's culinary roots. It's perfect for those who appreciate bold and unique flavors.

Lamington with Popcorn

Lamington is a cherished Australian dessert of sponge cake coated in chocolate and coconut which is loved by almost everyone in the country. Thus, many have tried incorporating popcorn into this delightful treat. This sweet creation combines chocolate and coconut flavors with the satisfying crunch of popcorn, resulting in a delicious snack that captures the essence of the much-adored dessert. It showcases Australia's enthusiasm for inventive and indulgent treats while offering a taste of the nation's culinary essence.

New Zealand

Hokey Pokey Popcorn

Drawing inspiration from the classic New Zealand ice cream flavor, hokey pokey, made with caramelized sugar and baking soda, hokey pokey popcorn delivers a delightful taste of this iconic sweet. The blend of crunchy popcorn and sweet, toffee-like hokey pokey flavors creates an enticing snack that reflects New Zealand's fondness for sugary treats. This popcorn variety emphasizes the creative fusion of flavors that characterizes the country's culinary traditions, providing a scrumptious insight into its unique confections.

Manuka honey popcorn

Manuka honey, native to New Zealand, is renowned for its rich flavor and unique health benefits. Drawing inspiration from this treasured ingredient, Manuka honey popcorn combines the delicate sweetness of Manuka honey with the satisfying crunch of popcorn, resulting in a delightful and wholesome treat. This popcorn creation highlights the importance of local ingredients in New Zealand's culinary culture and offers a delicious taste of the country's rich natural resources.

The diverse culinary landscape of Oceania has inspired a variety of unique and delicious popcorn flavors that pay tribute to the region's rich cultural traditions. By incorporating iconic ingredients and flavors from Australia and New Zealand, these popcorn creations showcase the distinct character of each country, providing snackers with a taste of Oceania's vibrant culinary scene. With the bold, savory flavors of Vegemite popcorn to the sweet treat of hokey pokey popcorn, these popcorn varieties highlight Oceania's creative flair and passion for food/ Thus, giving a delectable peek into the region's distinctive culinary traditions.

Middle East

The Middle East boasts a diverse culinary landscape as it is shaped by its rich heritage. Aside from this, it is known for its use of remarkable spices, flavors, and ingredients that make its cuisine truly unique. As a result, an array of popcorn variations has emerged, highlighting the distinct tastes of this captivating region. From the luxurious saffron-infused popcorn in Iran to the sweet Turkish delight popcorn, these creations offer a window into the diverse flavors of the Middle East.

Iran

Saffron-infused popcorn

Drawing inspiration from Iran's love for saffron, a precious and fragrant spice, saffron-infused popcorn highlights the delicate, floral taste of this cherished ingredient. The combination of crunchy popcorn and luxurious saffron creates a unique and sophisticated snack that pays homage to Iran's rich culinary culture and love for refined flavors.

Pomegranate and Rosewater Popcorn

Taking cues from the lively flavors of Iran, pomegranate and rosewater popcorn melds the sweet-sour taste of pomegranate with the gentle, floral notes of rosewater. This delightful popcorn creation highlights the balance of flavors found in Iranian cuisine, offering a scrumptious taste of the nation's rich culinary heritage.

Turkey

Turkish Delight Popcorn

Turkish delight, a treasured confection in Turkey, has sparked the idea for a one-of-a-kind popcorn flavor. Brands such as Uniqourn have embraced this flavor profile and crafted a popcorn mix that presents a sweet and fragrant snack reminiscent of the classic treat. By merging flavors like rose, lemon, and pomegranate with the satisfying crunch of popcorn, Turkish delight, popcorn serves as a delightful tribute to Turkey's love for distinctive and indulgent sweets.

Olive Oil and Thyme Popcorn

Influenced by the Mediterranean elements in Turkish cuisine, olive oil, and thyme popcorn fuses the earthy, aromatic flavors of thyme with the lushness of olive oil. This popcorn creation highlights the diverse flavors that define Turkey's culinary scene and offers a singular taste of the country's flavorful and aromatic dishes.

Israel

Za'atar-Spiced Popcorn

Taking cues from the much-loved Middle Eastern spice blend known as za'atar, za'atar-spiced popcorn combines the flavors of thyme, sumac, and sesame seeds to create a tasty and aromatic treat that everyone can savor. This popcorn variety showcases the unique tastes of Israeli cuisine, emphasizing the bold and fragrant flavors that characterize the region's culinary traditions.

Tahini-Drizzled Popcorn

Tahini, a sesame seed paste, plays a crucial role in Israeli cuisine and has inspired the scrumptious creation of tahini-drizzled popcorn. Combining the nutty, creamy flavor of tahini with the satisfying crunch of popcorn results in a delectable and unique snack that celebrates Israel's culinary traditions and the significance of sesame seeds in the nation's food scene.

Lebanon

Sumac and Lemon Popcorn

Lebanon's love for tangy and zesty flavors has led to the creation of sumac and lemon popcorn, a unique snack that blends the tartness of sumac with the bright, citrusy notes of lemon. This popcorn variety offers a delicious taste of Lebanon's culinary traditions, showcasing the bold and vibrant flavors that characterize the country's cuisine.

United Arab Emirates

Cardamom and cinnamon popcorn

Drawing inspiration from the captivating aromas of the United Arab Emirates, cardamom and cinnamon popcorn blends these delightful spices, crafting a warm and alluring snack. This popcorn delight highlights the vibrant and exotic flavors that epitomize the UAE's culinary world, giving you a one-of-a-kind taste of the region's intricate and diverse spice medleys.

The Middle East's bountiful culinary history has sparked a variety of popcorn flavors that celebrate the unique tastes and ingredients found in this mesmerizing region. By infusing traditional spices, flavors, and native ingredients, these popcorn concoctions let you savor the wide-ranging culinary customs that define the Middle East. Ranging from the opulent saffron-laced popcorn of Iran to the aromatic cardamom and cinnamon popcorn from the United Arab Emirates, these inventive popcorn flavors provide a distinctive and delectable glimpse into the area's rich cultural legacy.

Tips for Choosing the Perfect Popcorn Flavor: A Guide for Snack Enthusiasts

With the vast array of popcorn flavors available from around the world, choosing the perfect popcorn flavor can be an exciting but challenging task. In this section, discover helpful tips for selecting popcorn flavors that cater to individual tastes and preferences, ensuring a satisfying snacking experience.

Know Your Taste Preferences

- Sweet vs. savory: Determine whether you prefer sweet or savory flavors, as this will help narrow down your options when choosing a popcorn flavor.
- Spiciness: Consider your tolerance for spicy foods, as some popcorn flavors can pack quite a punch.
- Boldness: Some popcorn flavors can be quite bold and intense, while others are milder and more subtle. Know your preference for flavor intensity when selecting a popcorn variety.

Explore International Flavors

- Get inspired by global cuisines: If you enjoy exploring the flavors of different cultures, opt for popcorn flavors inspired by international dishes and ingredients. Don't forget to check out the various flavors we shared previously as you can taste the culinary richness of different countries and cuisines.
- Consider regional preferences: Keep in mind that some flavors may be more popular or readily available in certain regions, so consider your location when selecting a popcorn flavor. This applies if you are buying prepackaged popcorn. If ever you are making your own, there are also ingredients that are not readily available in your area. Don't worry! You just need to be creative when mixing and curating your own flavor.

Pairings and Occasions

- Match with beverages: Consider popcorn flavors that pair well with your favorite beverages, such as wine, beer, or soft drinks. For example, savory popcorn, such as the beloved cheddar cheese or the spice-heavy like Masala-flavored popcorn is perfect with soda.

Dietary Considerations

- Allergies and sensitivities: Be mindful of any food allergies or sensitivities when selecting popcorn flavors, as some may contain ingredients such as nuts or dairy. Take note that some popcorn uses milk and butter in their flavoring or there are also popcorn mixes that include a variety of nuts. For example, avoid the groundnut or peanut butter popcorn of Nigeria if you are allergic to peanuts.
- Health-conscious options: For those who prefer healthier snacks, look for popcorn flavors that are air-popped, low in sodium, and made with natural ingredients. An example of this is the olive oil and thyme flavor of Turkey.

Experiment and Have Fun

- Try new flavors: Don't be afraid to step outside your comfort zone and try new popcorn flavors. You might discover a new favorite!
- Create your own: Get creative in the kitchen and experiment with making your own popcorn flavors using spices, herbs, and other ingredients.

By following these tips, you can make better-informed decisions when selecting popcorn flavors that cater to your taste preferences and snacking needs. Keep in mind that everyone's palate is different, and part of the fun is discovering new and exciting flavors that you might enjoy.

Aside from this, don't hesitate to experiment with various popcorn types, whether they're sweet, savory, or something in between. By keeping an open mind and trying out diverse options, you'll not only broaden your snacking horizons but also develop a deeper appreciation for the wide-ranging world of popcorn. Remember, the key is to have fun while exploring different flavors and finding your personal favorites!

The world of popcorn is a fascinating and diverse realm of flavors, popping methods, and consumption styles. As we have explored the various ways in which popcorn is enjoyed across different countries and continents, it is evident that this simple yet versatile snack transcends cultural boundaries and unites people through a shared love for its delightful taste and texture. From the classic buttery popcorn of the United States to the exotic saffron-infused popcorn of Iran, these unique flavors showcase the rich culinary heritage and creativity of different regions around the globe.

Remember to keep an open mind, embrace new tastes, and have fun experimenting with different flavor combinations when trying out new popcorn flavors. Whether you prefer the sweet and comforting taste of caramel corn or the bold and savory kick of masala popcorn, there is a popcorn variety out there to suit every palate. Don't be afraid to go out of your comfort zone and try the flavors we've listed down for you. Experience different culinary flavors just by eating a simple but delicious popcorn snack.

Chapter 8

Types of Poppers

The magic of popcorn lies in the remarkable transformation of simple corn kernels into a fluffy and irresistible snack. This culinary marvel occurs when the kernel expands rapidly upon heating, turning the moisture inside into steam and producing the characteristic "pop" sound. Achieving this delightful outcome requires just the right blend of heat and pressure.

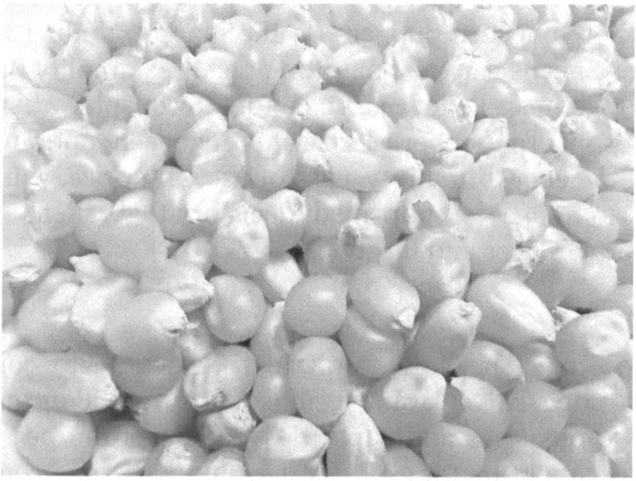

This is where a popcorn popper is important. It is a specialized appliance designed to create the perfect environment for popcorn popping. They guarantee that each kernel reaches its full potential, resulting in a light and airy snack with minimal waste through evenly distributing heat and maintaining the ideal temperature. With a wide range of popcorn poppers to suit various tastes and needs, you're sure to find the perfect option for a quick and simple snack or a more elaborate popcorn experience.

In this chapter, we will discuss the factors to consider when choosing the perfect popcorn popper for your needs. We'll also explore the pros and cons of different types of popcorn poppers, such as air poppers, stovetop poppers, electric poppers, microwave poppers, commercial popcorn machines, and campfire popcorn makers. Plus, we'll touch on popcorn popper accessories, maintenance, and safety to give you a well-rounded understanding of these appliances.

By the end of this chapter, you'll have the knowledge to make an informed choice about the best popcorn popper for your unique preferences. Whether you're a casual popcorn fan or a devoted enthusiast, our mission is to enhance your popcorn experience by helping you find the perfect machine to pop your delicious snacks. So, let's embark on this exciting journey together and discover the ultimate tool for creating your favorite fluffy snack.

Criteria for Choosing the Right Popcorn Popper

With so many popcorn poppers on the market, finding the perfect one for your needs can be a daunting task. To simplify the process, we've put together a list of crucial factors to consider when selecting the ideal popcorn popper. By evaluating each option based on capacity, efficiency, durability, ease of use, and price, you'll be well-equipped to make an informed decision that aligns with your snacking preferences and lifestyle.

Capacity

When choosing a popcorn popper, it's essential to consider the amount of popcorn you want to make at a time. Popcorn poppers come in various sizes and capacities, ranging from personal-sized portions to larger quantities fit for a group. Assessing your popcorn consumption habits will help you determine the ideal capacity for your needs.

For instance, if you typically make popcorn for family movie nights or gatherings, a larger capacity popper may be a better choice. On the other hand, if you usually enjoy popcorn as a solo snack, a smaller capacity popper might be more suitable. Keep in mind that some models are more versatile, offering adjustable capacities to cater to different situations. Examples of popcorn poppers with varying capacities include a hand crank stovetop popper, which can make up to 6 quarts of popcorn, and the Cuisinart EasyPop hot air popcorn maker, suitable for making smaller portions.

Efficiency

Efficiency is another critical factor when selecting a popcorn popper. An efficient popper will consistently produce perfectly popped kernels with minimal waste. Look for models that can achieve a high popping ratio, leaving very few un-popped kernels behind.

Heat distribution plays a significant role in a popcorn popper's efficiency. Look for poppers that ensure even heat distribution, allowing all the kernels to pop uniformly. Additionally, consider the popping speed of the popper. Some models can make a batch of popcorn in just a few minutes, while others may take longer. For example, the Presto PopLite hot air popper boasts a rapid popping time of 2.5 minutes for a 12-cup batch, making it an efficient choice for those who value speed.

Durability

Durability is a crucial consideration when investing in a popcorn popper. A well-built and durable popper will provide years of reliable service, offering excellent value for your money. Look for models constructed with high-quality materials, such as stainless steel or heavy-duty plastic, to ensure longevity.

Pay attention to the warranty provided by the manufacturer, as this can be an indicator of the popper's expected durability. A longer warranty period typically signifies that the manufacturer has confidence in the product's quality and lifespan. For example, the Great Northern Popcorn Company's stainless steel stovetop popper comes with a 5-year warranty, showcasing the manufacturer's commitment to the product's durability.

Ease of Use

A popcorn popper should be easy to use, allowing you to make delicious popcorn with minimal effort. User-friendly features, such as clear instructions, simple controls, and easy assembly, can make your popcorn-making experience more enjoyable. Assess the ease of adding kernels and other ingredients, as well as the convenience of monitoring the popping process.

Some popcorn poppers, like the Ecolution Original Microwave Micro-Pop popcorn popper, come with a built-in measuring cup and require no oil, making it incredibly simple to use. Others, like the West Bend Stir Crazy electric popcorn popper, feature a motorized stirring rod that ensures even popping without manual intervention.

Price

Finally, you should consider the price of the popcorn popper in relation to your budget and the features it offers. It's essential to compare and contrast the cost and quality when it may be tempting to opt for the cheapest option available. Keep in mind that a higher-priced popper may offer better durability, efficiency, and performance, providing better value in the long run.

When evaluating the price of a popcorn popper, consider the cost of ownership as well. This is more important for those who will be selling popcorn as this includes expenses related to maintenance, replacement parts, and accessories, such as popcorn kernels, oil, and seasoning. For example, hot air poppers may be more affordable in the long run due to their oil-free operation, which reduces the overall cost of making popcorn.

To find the best popcorn popper within your budget, compare models based on their features, performance, and user reviews. This will help you identify a popper that offers the best value for your money while meeting your popcorn-making needs.

In conclusion, choosing the right popcorn popper involves carefully evaluating the capacity, efficiency, durability, ease of use, and price of each model. By considering these criteria and comparing various options, you can find the perfect popcorn popper to satisfy your cravings and enhance your popcorn experience. Whether you're a casual snacker or a true popcorn aficionado, investing in the right popcorn popper will bring the joy of perfectly popped, delicious popcorn into your home.

Types of Popcorn Poppers

There are several types of popcorn poppers with different methods of popping kernels. This is important to take note of since they each deliver a distinctive popcorn experience. In this section, we will explore the popular popcorn poppers. We will discuss how they work, their advantages and disadvantages, their best uses and some popular models on the market.

Stove Top

Using a pot to make stove-top popcorn is a time-honored method that conjures up nostalgic memories of cozy movie nights and the intoxicating aroma of freshly popped corn. While this approach certainly has its advantages, it also comes with its own set of disadvantages. In this exploration, we'll delve into the perks, drawbacks, and best uses of making stove-top popcorn with a trusty pot.

Advantages

Cost-Effective: One of the most significant advantages of using a pot to make popcorn is its cost-effectiveness. Most households already have a suitable pot in their kitchen, eliminating the need for additional equipment or specialized popcorn makers. This makes stove-top popcorn an economical choice.

Customization: When you make popcorn in a pot, you have complete control over the ingredients and flavors. You can experiment with various oils (like coconut, olive, or ghee) and seasonings (such as salt, nutritional yeast, or herbs) to create a personalized popcorn experience that suits your taste preferences.

No Microwave Required: For those without access to a microwave or who prefer to avoid microwaveable bags due to health concerns, stove-top popcorn offers a convenient alternative. All you need is a stovetop, a pot with a lid, and some popcorn kernels.

Better Flavor and Texture: Stove-top popcorn often boasts superior flavor and texture compared to microwave varieties. The direct heat from the stovetop encourages even popping and allows for a more authentic popcorn experience, with a delightful mix of crunchy and fluffy kernels.

Fun and Engaging: Making popcorn in a pot can be a fun and engaging activity for kids and adults alike. The anticipation of waiting for the first pop, the sounds of kernels popping, and the ultimate satisfaction of creating a snack from scratch can be a delightful experience.

Disadvantages

Requires Close Monitoring: Making popcorn in a pot requires vigilant attention. You must continuously shake or stir the pot to prevent kernels from burning or sticking to the bottom. This hands-on approach can be time-consuming and demanding.

Risk of Burnt Kernels: Without proper timing and attention, it's easy to burn some of the kernels in the pot. Burnt popcorn can impart an unpleasant, bitter taste to the entire batch.

Potential Mess: Stove-top popcorn can sometimes be messier than using microwaveable bags. Popped kernels may scatter, leaving behind un-popped ones and oily residue on the stovetop and surrounding areas.

Inconsistent Results: Achieving consistently perfect popcorn can be challenging when using a pot. Factors like the pot's size, lid design, and heat source can lead to variations in popping efficiency and kernel distribution.

Best Uses

Snack Time: Stove-top popcorn is an ideal choice for snack time, whether you're enjoying a family movie night or a casual evening with friends. Its versatility allows you to tailor the flavors to your liking.

Healthy Snacking: If you're health-conscious, stove-top popcorn offers a healthier alternative to pre-packaged, heavily processed snacks. You can control the type and amount of oil and seasonings, making it a nutritious choice.

Flavor Experimentation: Stove-top popcorn is a canvas for culinary creativity. Experiment with different oils, herbs, spices, and even sweeteners like honey or maple syrup to create unique flavor profiles.

Cooking with Kids: Making popcorn in a pot can be a delightful cooking activity for children, teaching them about kitchen safety, patience, and the transformation of raw ingredients into a tasty treat.

Using a pot to make stove-top popcorn offers a cost-effective and customizable snack-making experience with superior flavor and texture. While it may require close monitoring and comes with the risk of burning kernels, it remains a beloved method for creating a classic snack. Whether for movie nights, healthy snacking, flavor experimentation, or as a fun cooking activity with kids, stove-top popcorn continues to pop its way into our hearts and homes.

Air Popper

Air poppers are a popular and healthy way to enjoy popcorn, as they do not require any oil for the popping process. Instead, they rely on hot air circulation to heat the kernels evenly and quickly. The air popper's design features a small heating element at the bottom of the unit, surrounded by vents that allow hot air to flow into the popping chamber. As the hot air circulates, the kernels are agitated and heated until they reach the perfect temperature to pop. Once the popcorn has popped, the lightweight, fluffy kernels are blown out of the chamber and into a waiting bowl.

Advantages

One of the most significant advantages of air poppers is their ability to produce oil-free popcorn, resulting in a healthier and lower-calorie snack. This makes them an excellent choice for those watching their calorie intake or looking to enjoy popcorn without added fat.

Air poppers are also known for their speed and efficiency, often popping kernels in just a few minutes. The hot air circulation ensures even heat distribution, reducing the number of un-popped kernels left behind. Additionally, air poppers are typically compact and easy to store, making them suitable for small kitchens or limited counter space.

Disadvantages

Despite their many advantages, air poppers do have some drawbacks. Because they rely on hot air to pop the kernels, the popcorn produced can sometimes be drier and less flavorful compared to popcorn made with oil. However, this can be remedied by adding your choice of seasoning or a light spray of oil after popping.

Air poppers can also be somewhat noisy during operation, as the hot air circulation creates a loud whirring sound. Lastly, some users have reported that air poppers can blow un-popped kernels out of the chamber along with the popped popcorn. Placing a larger bowl around the popper or using a kernel catcher can help minimize this issue.

Best Uses

Opt for an air popper if you are looking for a quick, convenient, and healthy way to enjoy popcorn at home. This is because are ideal for people who prefer oil-free popcorn and are watching their calorie intake. It could also be for those who want to simply enjoy the taste and texture of air-popped popcorn. Additionally, air poppers are also a great option for those with limited kitchen space, as they are compact and easy to store.

Popular Air Popper Models

Presto PopLite Hot Air Popper: This popular model is known for its speed, popping kernels in under 2.5 minutes. It is also known for its compact design and is available in multiple colors.

Cuisinart EasyPop Hot Air Popcorn Maker: Featuring a removable chute and butter warming tray, this air popper allows for easy customization of your popcorn with your choice of seasoning or butter.

There are even commercial air poppers you can buy which is a great healthy base for flavoring popcorn.

Electric Popcorn Popper

Electric popcorn poppers combine the convenience of an air popper with the traditional oil-popping method found in stovetop poppers. These poppers feature an electric heating element that heats the oil and kernels, causing them to pop. Most electric popcorn poppers have a built-in stirring mechanism that keeps the kernels moving to ensure even heat distribution and prevent burning. To use an electric popcorn popper, simply add oil and popcorn kernels to the popping chamber, plug the unit in, and turn it on. Once the popping process is complete, the popped popcorn is ready to be seasoned and enjoyed.

Advantages

Electric popcorn poppers offer several advantages, such as consistent and even heat distribution, resulting in fewer un-popped kernels and a uniformly cooked batch of popcorn. They also provide a more hands-off approach compared to stovetop poppers, as the built-in stirring mechanism eliminates the need for manual stirring.

Another advantage of electric popcorn poppers is their versatility. They can be used with various oils and seasonings, allowing for a wide range of popcorn flavors and textures. Some models even come with a built-in butter dispenser, making it easy to add your desired amount of melted butter to your popcorn.

Disadvantages

One notable disadvantage of electric popcorn poppers is their reliance on electricity, which may not be ideal for those who prefer energy-efficient appliances or want to minimize their energy consumption. Additionally, electric poppers can be bulkier and take up more counter space than other types of popcorn poppers.

Cleaning electric popcorn poppers can also be more challenging, as some models may not have removable parts or may require careful cleaning around the heating element. Furthermore, electric popcorn poppers tend to be more expensive than air poppers or stovetop models, making them a more significant investment.

Best Uses

Electric popcorn poppers are ideal for those who want a convenient and hands-off method of making popcorn while still enjoying the traditional oil-popped flavor and texture. They are well-suited for family movie nights, parties, or other occasions where large batches of popcorn are needed quickly and with minimal effort. Electric poppers are also a good option for those who enjoy experimenting with different oils and seasonings, as they offer greater versatility than air poppers.

Popular Electric Popcorn Popper Models

West Bend Stir Crazy Electric Popcorn Popper: This popular model features a non-stick popping surface, a built-in stirring mechanism, and a vented lid that doubles as a serving bowl.

Nostalgia Vintage Collection Electric Popcorn Popper: Designed with a retro aesthetic, this popper has a large 2.5-ounce stainless steel kettle and a built-in stirring system, perfect for making popcorn with a nostalgic touch.

Microwave Popcorn Popper

Microwave popcorn poppers are designed to be used in a microwave oven, offering a quick and convenient method of making popcorn at home. These poppers are typically made of microwave-safe materials, such as silicone or heat-resistant plastic, and have a vented lid that allows steam to escape during the popping process. To use a microwave popcorn popper, simply add popcorn kernels and oil (if desired) to the popper, place the lid on top, and set it in the microwave. The cooking time will vary depending on the microwave's power and the amount of popcorn being made, but most microwave poppers can produce a batch of popcorn in just a few minutes.

Advantages

Microwave popcorn poppers offer several advantages, including speed and convenience. They can quickly produce popcorn using a microwave, eliminating the need for additional appliances or stovetop use. Microwave poppers also provide flexibility in terms of oil use; you can opt for oil-free popcorn or add your preferred oil for a richer flavor.

Another advantage of microwave popcorn poppers is their easy cleanup. Many models are dishwasher safe or can be easily washed by hand, making them low-maintenance options for busy households. Finally, microwave poppers are often compact and easy to store, making them an excellent choice for those with limited kitchen space.

Disadvantages

A significant issue with microwave poppers is that they depend on the microwave's power and performance. Microwaves can greatly differ in efficiency, which might lead to uneven cooking or a higher number of un-popped kernels in some cases. Additionally, microwave poppers may not be as durable as other types since they're often made from lighter materials like silicone or plastic.

Another disadvantage of microwave poppers is the limited control over the cooking process. Unlike other popcorn makers, you may not have much room for adjusting temperature or cooking time, which could impact the quality of your popcorn. Nevertheless, despite these potential drawbacks, microwave poppers remain a handy and quick option for those craving a delicious snack without too much fuss.

Best Uses

Microwave popcorn poppers are perfect for those seeking a quick, hassle-free, and low-maintenance way to whip up popcorn at home. They're an excellent choice for on-the-go individuals, college students, or anyone working with limited kitchen space or appliances. Microwave poppers cater to various preferences, offering the flexibility to make popcorn with or without oil, making them a versatile option for diverse snacking styles. So, if you're after an easy and adaptable method to satisfy your popcorn cravings, microwave popcorn poppers might just be the right choice for you.

Popular Microwave Popcorn Popper Models

Lekue Microwave Popcorn Popper: Made from BPA-free platinum silicone, this collapsible popper is dishwasher safe and can produce up to 10 cups of popcorn in just a few minutes.

Nordic Ware Microwave Popcorn Popper: This versatile popper, made from BPA-free and melamine-free plastic, can also be used on the stovetop for those who prefer traditional cooking methods.

<u>Commercial Popcorn Machine</u>

Commercial popcorn machines are expertly designed to churn out heaps of popcorn in bustling places like movie theaters, concession stands, and big events. These machines typically have a large stainless steel or aluminum kettle, which is warmed by an electric or gas-powered heating element. To whip up some popcorn, simply pour oil and kernels into the kettle, switch on the machine, and let the oil heat up. As the kernels get toasty, they start to pop and soon get released into the surrounding chamber, making it super easy to serve.

Most commercial popcorn machines come with a built-in stirring mechanism to avoid burning and promote even cooking. Some models also include features like a warming deck to keep the popcorn fresh and toasty, a built-in butter dispenser for easy flavoring, and tempered glass windows so you can watch the popping process.

Advantages

One of the main advantages of commercial popcorn machines is their ability to produce large quantities of popcorn quickly and efficiently. Thus, making them ideal for high-demand environments. They are also built to withstand heavy use, with durable materials and high-quality components ensuring long-lasting performance.

Aside from this, offer consistency in the popping process due to their precise temperature controls and even heat distribution. This results in a high-quality product with fewer un-popped kernels. Additionally, the eye-catching design of these machines can boost the ambiance of an event or venue, making them a popular choice for businesses and event planners.

Disadvantages

However, there are some downsides to commercial popcorn machines. Their primary drawback is their higher price point compared to other popcorn poppers. Moreover, they demand more space and might not be the best choice for home use or smaller events due to their size and power requirements.

Another potential disadvantage is the maintenance and cleaning associated with these machines. Regular cleaning is crucial to avoid oil and residue buildup, which could affect the machine's performance and lifespan. Furthermore, commercial machines might call for more specialized care and maintenance compared to smaller, home-use poppers. Despite these drawbacks, commercial popcorn machines remain an attractive option for those looking to provide a memorable popcorn experience on a larger scale.

Best Uses

Commercial popcorn machines are perfect for large-scale events, movie theaters, concession stands, and other busy locations where producing substantial amounts of popcorn is necessary. Businesses like rental companies, catering services, and event planners can also take advantage of these machines, as they offer a dependable and efficient way to make popcorn for various occasions.

Popular Commercial Popcorn Machine Models

Gold Medal Pop Maxx Popcorn Machine: This high-capacity machine comes with a 12- or 14-ounce kettle, a heated corn deck, and a built-in exhaust system, ensuring the popcorn stays fresh and warm.

Paragon Theater Pop Popcorn Machine: Available in multiple kettle sizes, this model features a durable anodized aluminum kettle, a warming deck, and a presentation lamp for a visually appealing display.

Campfire Popcorn Maker

Campfire popcorn makers are designed for outdoor use, allowing you to make popcorn over an open fire or a portable camping stove. These typically consist of a long handle with a heat-resistant grip and a popping chamber and are made of sturdy materials such as stainless steel, cast iron, or aluminum. To use this kind of popper, simply add oil and kernels to the popping chamber, close the lid or cover, and hold it over the heat source. As its contents heat up, they pop and fill the chamber. Once the popping is done, remove the popper from the heat, open the lid, and serve the warm and delicious popcorn.

Advantages

One of the main advantages of campfire popcorn makers is their portability, making them an excellent choice for outdoor enthusiasts and campers who want to enjoy freshly made popcorn while in the great outdoors. These popcorn makers are lightweight, compact, and easy to pack, ensuring minimal impact on your camping gear.

Campfire popcorn makers also provide a fun and interactive cooking experience, allowing you to engage with the popping process and enjoy the sights and sounds of making popcorn over an open flame. This can be an enjoyable activity for families and groups of friends during camping trips or backyard bonfires.

Another advantage of campfire popcorn makers is their durability. Many models are made from sturdy materials like cast iron or stainless steel, which can withstand high temperatures and resist rust and corrosion.

Disadvantages

One of the main disadvantages of campfire popcorn makers is the reliance on an open flame or heat source, which can be challenging to control and maintain, especially in windy or damp conditions. This may result in uneven cooking or a higher number of un-popped kernels.

Campfire popcorn makers may also require more attention and manual effort compared to other types of popcorn poppers, as you need to continuously shake or move the popper over the heat source to ensure even heat distribution and prevent burning.

Another potential drawback of campfire popcorn makers is their limited batch size. Due to their compact design, these popcorn makers generally produce smaller quantities of popcorn per batch compared to other types of popcorn poppers.

Best Uses

This type of popper is perfect for someone who enjoys spending time in the great outdoors, whether you are camping, having a picnic, or just sitting around a backyard bonfire, it's the ideal way to enjoy fresh, hot popcorn. However, it is also great for any occasion where you have access to an open flame or portable heat source.

Popular Campfire Popcorn Maker

Hand Crank Campfire Popper: What makes this popcorn maker stand out is it is made of high-quality aluminum and has a patented stirring mechanism that ensures all the kernels are popped evenly.

Rome's Popcorn Popper: This popcorn maker is made of heavy-duty steel and has a non-stick cooking surface that makes cleaning a breeze. It also comes with a long handle that stays cool to the touch and has a comfortable grip.

Extra Popcorn Popper Accessories

To make your popcorn-making experience even better and more convenient, there are a variety of popcorn popper accessories available to help you prepare, serve, and store your popcorn effortlessly. Here are some popular accessories you might want to consider:

Popcorn Scoops

Popcorn scoops are handy tools for transferring freshly popped popcorn from the popper to serving bowls or bags without making a mess. They come in various sizes and materials such as plastic, aluminum, or stainless steel, ensuring you can find the perfect scoop for your needs.

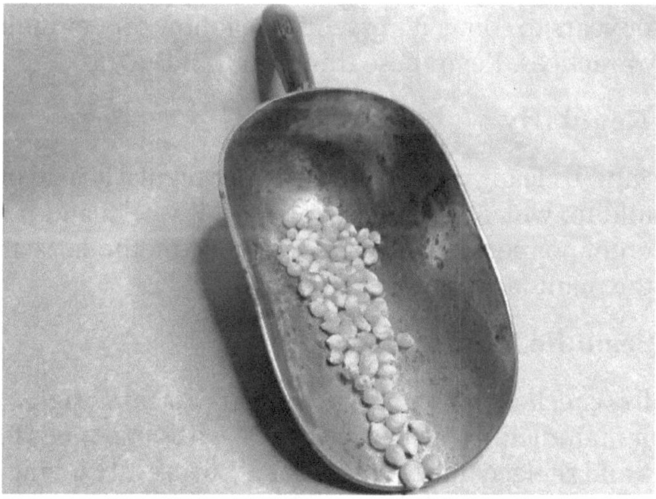

Popcorn Scoop

Butter Dispensers

Butter dispensers allow you to add the perfect amount of melted butter to your popcorn with ease. Available in manual pump or electric models, these dispensers can be placed on your countertop, making it simple to drizzle butter over your popcorn for a delicious, movie theater-style treat.

Seasoning Shakers

Seasoning shakers are perfect for adding a burst of flavor to your popcorn. They come in various designs and sizes, with pre-filled options or empty containers to fill with your favorite seasonings. From classic salt and butter to more adventurous flavors, seasoning shakers make customizing your popcorn a breeze.

Storage Containers

Proper storage containers help keep your popcorn fresh and crisp for longer periods. Airtight containers, resealable bags, or specially designed popcorn storage tins can all help preserve the freshness and taste of your popcorn, ensuring you can enjoy delicious, homemade popcorn whenever the craving strikes.

Popcorn Popper Maintenance and Safety

To ensure the longevity of your popcorn popper and enjoy delicious popcorn for years to come, it's essential to follow proper maintenance and safety practices. Keep these things in mind:

Clean It Regularly

It's important to clean your popcorn popper regularly to avoid oil and residue buildup, which can affect how well it works and how long it lasts. Different poppers need specific cleaning methods, so make sure to follow the manufacturer's instructions.

Ensure Periodic Maintenance

Periodically check your popcorn popper for any signs of wear, damage, or malfunction. Inspect electrical cords and plugs for fraying or damage and replace them if necessary. Ensure all moving parts are functioning smoothly and lubricate them as needed.

Store It Properly

Proper storage of your popcorn popper is essential to protect it from dust, moisture, and damage. Regardless of the type, store your poppers in a cool, dry place away from direct sunlight and extreme temperatures. If applicable, Keep the power cord neatly wrapped to avoid damage. You can keep them in a cabinet or pantry, ensuring they're clean and dry before putting it away. Lastly, avoid stacking heavy items on top of the popper to prevent damage.

Safety Tips

Following safety guidelines when using your popcorn popper can prevent accidents and ensure a pleasant popcorn-making experience. Here are some general safety tips:

- Always follow the manufacturer's instructions for use and care.
- Unplug electric popcorn poppers before cleaning or when not in use.
- Do not immerse electrical appliances in water or any other liquid.
- Use heat-resistant oven mitts or potholders when handling hot popcorn poppers.
- Keep children and pets away from hot popcorn poppers.
- Never leave a popcorn popper unattended while in use.
- Avoid overfilling popcorn poppers with kernels, as this can lead to uneven cooking or damage to the popper.
- Do not use damaged or malfunctioning popcorn poppers.

Throughout this chapter, we have explored the various types of popcorn poppers, from air poppers and stovetop poppers to electric poppers, microwave poppers, and commercial popcorn machines. We've also delved into the world of campfire popcorn makers for those who prefer a more nostalgic and interactive popcorn-making experience. By examining the advantages and disadvantages of each type, we hope that this information provided you with the knowledge you need to find the perfect popper for your specific requirements.

As you embark on your popcorn-popping journey, remember that the perfect popcorn popper is the one that best aligns with your unique needs and preferences. Whether you're searching for a compact microwave popper for quick snacking or a commercial machine to cater to large events, there's an option out there for everyone. Armed with the knowledge gained from this comprehensive guide, you're now ready to dive into the delightful world of popcorn poppers and discover the ideal tool for creating your favorite fluffy treat.

So, go ahead and indulge in the simple joy of making and sharing popcorn with friends and family, using the perfect popcorn popper to create unforgettable memories and mouthwatering snacks. Here's too many happy and delicious popcorn-filled moments!

Chapter 9

History of Poppers

Popcorn, a timeless snack enjoyed for centuries, traces its origins back to the indigenous peoples of the Americas. Its popularity has grown throughout the years, and today, it is an iconic treat in American culture and beyond. Popcorn poppers have played a vital role in making this classic snack more accessible and convenient to prepare. They have evolved from ancient techniques to modern appliances, providing a means to create the perfect pop with ease. Popcorn poppers are now a staple in households, movie theaters, and events, symbolizing togetherness and enjoyment across generations and cultures. The journey of popcorn poppers is a fascinating story of innovation, adaptation, and technology. Starting with clay pots and hot sand, popcorn-popping methods have progressed from fireplace cooking with long-handled pans to the sleek and efficient machines we know today. These advancements have made it possible for millions of people worldwide to indulge in the simple pleasure of freshly popped corn.

Early Popcorn Popping Methods: Native American Techniques

The fascinating journey of popcorn popping began thousands of years ago with the ingenious techniques of the indigenous peoples of the Americas. Among their various methods for turning hard corn kernels into a delightful snack, one stood out for its simplicity and effectiveness: using clay pots and hot sand. This early technique not only highlights the resourcefulness of these ancient cultures but also serves as the foundation upon which future popcorn-popping methods would be built.

Clay Pots and Hot Sand

Another early popcorn popping technique employed by Native Americans, which varied from tribe to tribe, likely originated from accidental discoveries. It is believed that some of the earliest popcorn enthusiasts may have thrown kernels into the fire and then eaten the popcorn as it popped and flew out of the flames. Historical evidence of more sophisticated popping methods comes from the Incas, whose ruins contain specially shaped clay pots with kernels of popped corn still inside them. This suggests a more refined approach to popcorn popping among certain Native American tribes.

The Incas' method involved heating sand and placing it in their unique clay pots, followed by scattering corn kernels on top of the sand. The pot was then covered with the heat from the sand causing the corn to pop. During the process, the heavier sand would remain at the bottom of the pot, while the popped kernels would rise above it, making them easily accessible. This method was ideal for outdoor gatherings, where participants could enjoy the delicious snack while engaging in social and ceremonial events.

Colonial Era Methods

As European settlers arrived in the Americas in the 16th and 17th centuries, they discovered popcorn and were introduced to this delightful snack by Native Americans. The colonists quickly adopted popcorn as part of their own culinary traditions, developing new methods to cook it that were better suited to their lifestyles and available tools.

Fireplace and Long-Handled Pans

The fireplace became the go-to method for popcorn popping in the colonial era. Long-handled pans with lids were used to cook the kernels over an open flame. The colonists would hold the pan above the fire, shaking it gently to ensure even heat distribution and to prevent the popcorn from burning. As the kernels heated up, they would burst open and fill the pan, creating a warm and inviting snack that was perfect for social gatherings and special occasions.

Wire Popcorn Poppers

The wire popcorn popper, a more advanced tool compared to the long-handled pan, also made its debut during the colonial era. This ingenious device featured a wire basket with a long handle, enabling users to hold it over an open flame without getting too close to the heat. The basket's design facilitated better air circulation, minimizing the chances of burnt popcorn and making it simpler to achieve a consistent pop.

Wire popcorn poppers were not just more efficient, but also highly versatile. They could be used over a fireplace or a campfire, becoming a popular option for outdoor events and gatherings. As popcorn gained popularity, the wire popcorn popper turned into a household essential in many colonial homes, setting the stage for future innovations in popcorn popping technology.

The Emergence of Modern Popcorn Popping Techniques

The early popcorn-popping methods used by Native Americans and colonial settlers may seem rudimentary compared to today's advanced machines, but they were an essential steppingstone in the evolution of popcorn poppers. The journey from clay pots and stone hearths to fireplaces and wire popcorn poppers demonstrated the adaptability and ingenuity of various cultures as they sought to perfect the art of popcorn popping.

As technology continued to advance and societies became more industrialized, new methods emerged, pushing the boundaries of what was possible and revolutionizing the way people enjoyed this simple snack. The industrial revolution, in particular, played a crucial role in the development of modern popcorn poppers, as inventors and entrepreneurs sought to capitalize on the snack's growing popularity by creating machines that could produce it more efficiently and consistently.

The Industrial Revolution and Popcorn Poppers

The Industrial Revolution, a time of rapid technological advancements and societal change, brought about innovations that would forever alter the art of popcorn popping. Among these breakthroughs were steam-powered popcorn machines, which revolutionized the way this beloved snack was prepared and enjoyed. These innovative machines paved the way for a new era of popcorn production, making the treat more accessible and captivating to the masses.

Charles Cretors' Invention

The first steam-powered popcorn machine was invented and patented by Charles Cretors in the late 19th century. Cretors, a confectioner based in Chicago, noticed the increasing demand for popcorn and aimed to develop a machine that could produce the snack more efficiently and consistently compared to existing methods.

In 1893, Cretors unveiled his invention: a steam-powered, horse-drawn popcorn machine that could not only popcorn but also roast peanuts and brew coffee. The machine showcased an enclosed glass case, allowing customers to watch the popcorn-making process, adding a touch of entertainment to the snacking experience. This represented a significant departure from earlier methods, which often involved popping corn in large, open pans or wire baskets over an open flame.

Popcorn Wagons and Street Vendors

Cretors' steam-powered popcorn machine revolutionized the way popcorn was sold and consumed. The invention gave rise to the popularity of popcorn wagons, which became a common sight on city streets and at carnivals and fairs. These mobile popcorn vendors offered a convenient way for people to enjoy freshly popped corn while on the go or at public events.

These are still prevalent today and even reached their peak popularity in the early 20th century, as enterprising vendors sought to capitalize on the snack's growing popularity. They became an emblem of American street food culture, evoking nostalgia for a simpler time and capturing the entrepreneurial spirit that defined the era.

Electric Popcorn Machines

The introduction of electricity in the late 19th and early 20th centuries further accelerated the evolution of popcorn poppers. As electric power became more widely available, inventors and manufacturers saw an opportunity to create popcorn machines that were even more efficient and user-friendly than their steam-powered counterparts.

The first electric popcorn machines emerged in the early 1900s, offering a cleaner and more consistent method of popping corn. These machines featured electric heating elements that eliminated the need for open flames or steam power, reducing the risk of accidents and making the popcorn-making process more streamlined.

Advancements in Technology and Design

Over the years, electric popcorn machines underwent numerous improvements in both technology and design. One of the most significant advancements was the introduction of the "stirring rod" mechanism, which automatically agitated the kernels to ensure even heat distribution and prevent burning. This innovation greatly improved the quality of the popped corn, resulting in a more enjoyable snacking experience.

In addition to technological advancements, electric popcorn machines also evolved in terms of design. Early models were often large, bulky, and industrial-looking, reflecting the utilitarian nature of the machines. However, as electric popcorn machines became more commonplace, manufacturers began to place a greater emphasis on aesthetics, creating machines with sleeker designs and eye-catching features, such as colorful exteriors.

These design improvements not only made electric popcorn machines more visually appealing but also helped to enhance the overall popcorn-eating experience. As popcorn became increasingly associated with leisure and entertainment, the machines themselves evolved into works of art that captured the imagination of the public.

The electric popcorn machines of today bear little resemblance to their early predecessors, yet they share a common lineage that can be traced back to the steam-powered machines of the Industrial Revolution. The development of these machines reflects the human desire for innovation and progress, as well as our enduring love for the simple pleasure of freshly popped corn.

A Shift in the Popcorn Industry

The popularity of hot air popcorn poppers represented a significant shift in the history of popcorn poppers, as manufacturers and consumers alike began to prioritize health-conscious options. This shift led to the development of various air popper models, each offering unique features and benefits aimed at making popcorn preparation even easier and more enjoyable. As a result, the popcorn industry began to focus more on the health aspects of their products, promoting the benefits of air-popped popcorn and offering a wider range of healthier seasoning options.

The Ongoing Evolution of Popcorn Poppers

The emergence of hot air popcorn poppers is a testament to the ongoing evolution of popcorn poppers throughout history. As societal trends and consumer preferences continue to change, the popcorn industry has adapted and innovated to meet these demands. Today, hot air popcorn poppers remain a popular choice for health-conscious consumers, proving that the desire for a healthier, guilt-free snack option is not just a passing trend, but a lasting influence on the popcorn popper market.

The Enduring Appeal of Stovetop Popcorn Poppers

Despite the rapid advancements in technology and the convenience offered by microwave and air popcorn poppers, stovetop popcorn poppers have maintained their popularity among a dedicated group of popcorn enthusiasts. There are several reasons why this traditional method of popping corn has endured in an age of modern gadgets and appliances.

The Authentic Popcorn Experience

For many popcorn lovers, using a stovetop popper harkens back to the nostalgic and authentic popcorn-making experience. The process of manually shaking the popper over a flame, listening to the kernels pop, and savoring the aroma of freshly popped corn evokes memories of simpler times and cherished moments with family and friends. The stovetop method provides a hands-on approach to popcorn making that many find satisfying and enjoyable.

Superior Taste and Texture

Many stovetop popcorn aficionados claim that this method produces popcorn with a superior taste and texture compared to microwave or air-popped varieties. Cooking the kernels in a bit of oil on the stovetop results in a richer, more flavorful snack that closely resembles the taste of movie theater popcorn. Additionally, stovetop popping tends to result in fewer un-popped kernels and a more consistent texture, which adds to the appeal of this traditional method.

Customization and Control

Stovetop popcorn poppers offer a level of customization and control that is not always possible with microwave or air poppers. Users can easily adjust the amount of oil, salt, and other seasonings to suit their preferences, creating a personalized popcorn experience. The stovetop method also allows for more even heat distribution, reducing the likelihood of burnt or unevenly popped kernels.

Durability and Versatility

Many stovetop popcorn poppers are built to last, with durable materials like stainless steel and cast iron. These poppers can withstand high heat and frequent use, making them a worthwhile investment for those who enjoy homemade popcorn regularly. Additionally, their versatility allows them to be used on various heat sources, including gas, electric, and even campfire stoves, making them a popular choice for outdoor enthusiasts and those who appreciate the portability of their cookware.

The enduring appeal of stovetop popcorn poppers demonstrates that even in our technologically advanced world, there is still a place for tradition and the simple pleasures that come with it. The authentic experience, superior taste, and customization options offered by stovetop poppers have allowed them to maintain their popularity and hold a special place in the hearts of popcorn lovers worldwide.

It's remarkable to see the diverse and evolving progression of methods used to pop the delightful snack we all love - popcorn. Every era, from the time of Native Americans to the Golden Age of Cinema, has contributed its own unique innovations to the art of popcorn popping. The relentless quest for the perfect popcorn experience has given us a broad range of popping methods, each with its distinct charm and advantages.

The enduring appeal of popcorn poppers across various eras and cultures highlights the versatility and adaptability of this simple yet delightful treat. As we continue to innovate and discover new ways to enjoy popcorn, we also pay homage to the rich history and traditions that have shaped the popcorn poppers we know and love today.

As we look to the future, it is exciting to consider what new advancements and innovations await us in the world of popcorn popping. The history of popcorn poppers has shown us that our love for this delicious snack knows no bounds, and we will undoubtedly continue to find creative and exciting ways to make the popcorn experience even more enjoyable for generations to come.

Chapter 10

Types of Popcorn Kernels

Have you ever considered the diversity of popcorn kernels and their distinct attributes?

In this chapter, we'll delve into the various types of popcorn kernels and uncover what makes each one unique. So, prepare a bowl of your go-to popcorn, sit back, and join us as we go through this comprehensive list of popcorn kernels.

Yellow Popcorn Kernels

Yellow popcorn is the type of kernel most people encounter in grocery stores. Available in an array of sizes, these kernels typically yield larger, fluffy, and somewhat chewy popcorn. It is the quintessential choice for movie nights, as it's recognized for its iconic buttery-yellow color, delivering the classic taste and texture everyone adores.

White Popcorn Kernels

In contrast to yellow popcorn, white popcorn kernels are smaller and more tender. These kernels create a delicate, almost melt-in-your-mouth popcorn with a hint of sweetness. White popcorn is well-suited for those seeking a more sophisticated snacking experience, as it tends to be less chewy and features a thinner hull, resulting in fewer pieces getting caught between your teeth. White popcorn kernels are frequently featured in gourmet popcorn creations, as their delicate texture and flavor profile makes them perfect for blending with sweet or savory ingredients. If you're ready to elevate your popcorn experience, give white popcorn a try!

Mushroom Popcorn Kernels

Mushroom popcorn kernels distinguish themselves by producing round, ball-shaped popcorn, unlike the irregular, butterfly-shaped popcorn resulting from yellow and white kernels. Aptly named, these kernels pop into a shape that mirrors a mushroom, offering a more consistent appearance and a delightfully crunchy texture.

Mushroom popcorn is the preferred option for caramel corn, kettle corn, and various flavored popcorn treats. Its strong, durable structure ensures it can handle the weight of coatings and glazes without becoming soggy or losing its crunch. Moreover, the round shape of mushroom popcorn and the absence of protruding "wings" make it less susceptible to breakage during the coating process, leading to a more visually appealing finished product. These are the type of popcorn kernels we like to pop with because they are hearty and large.

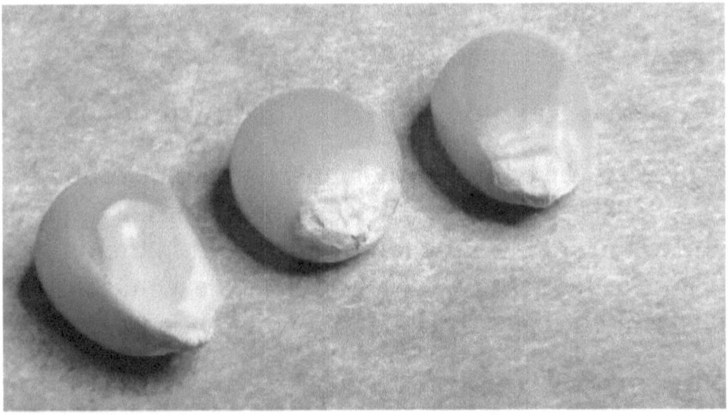

Mushroom Popcorn Kernels

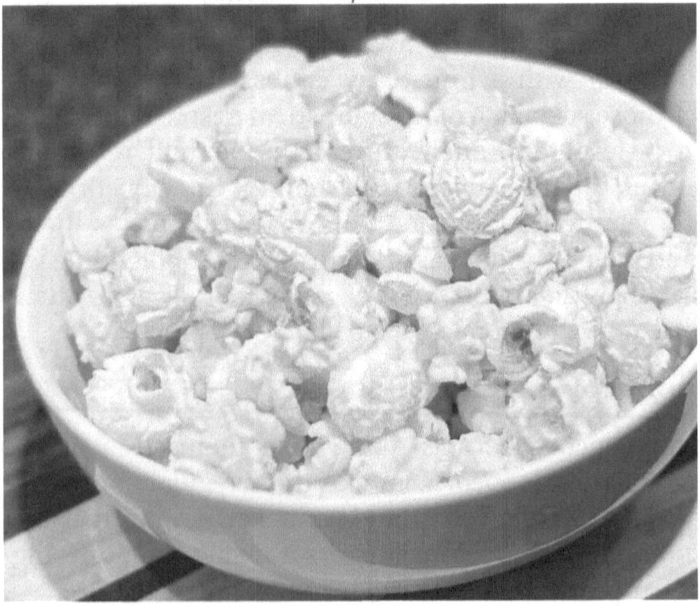

Popped Mushroom Kernels

Ladyfinger Kernels

Ladyfinger popcorn kernels are another unique variety worth exploring. These petite kernels produce small, tender popcorn with a delicate, almost hull-less texture. The name "ladyfinger" refers to the slender and elegant shape of the popped corn, which is reminiscent of the delicate cookies used in desserts such as tiramisu.

Ladyfinger popcorn is perfect for those who prefer a more refined snacking experience, as its tender texture and small size make it a delicate and delightful treat. This popcorn variety is also ideal for creating popcorn-based desserts and sweet treats, as its dainty size and shape lend themselves well to being combined with other ingredients like chocolate, nuts, and dried fruits.

Red Popcorn Kernels

Red popcorn kernels are a less common but visually striking option for popcorn enthusiasts. When popped, red popcorn kernels produce small to medium-sized popcorn with a subtly sweet, nutty flavor and a slightly crunchy texture. The red hue of the kernel is mostly lost during the popping process, but the resulting popcorn does retain a hint of a reddish tint.

Red popcorn kernels have a slightly higher nutritional content than their yellow and white counterparts, with increased levels of antioxidants thanks to their red pigmentation. This makes red popcorn a great choice for those seeking a healthier snacking option.

Blue Popcorn Kernels

Blue popcorn kernels stand out as a true gem in the popcorn universe. With their stunning blue hue, these kernels present a unique and eye-catching appearance. Once popped, blue popcorn kernels yield slightly smaller popcorn pieces with a tender, mildly sweet flavor, and a subtle blue tint.

Blue popcorn is packed with antioxidants, particularly anthocyanins, which are responsible for the kernel's blue color. This means that blue popcorn offers added health benefits compared to other popcorn varieties, making it an ideal choice for health-conscious snackers.

Black Popcorn Kernels

Black popcorn kernels are undoubtedly one of the most intriguing types of popcorn out there, and they're well worth a try. These kernels are characterized by their deep black color, which sets them apart from other popcorn varieties. Upon popping, black popcorn kernels reveal small, white popcorn pieces with a slightly nutty flavor and a pleasing crunch. Similar to blue popcorn, black popcorn is abundant in antioxidants due to the dark pigmentation of the kernels. This makes black popcorn another wholesome and tasty option for those seeking healthier snack alternatives.

Heirloom Popcorn Kernels

Heirloom popcorn kernels are varieties that have been passed down through generations, preserving their unique characteristics and avoiding the genetic modifications found in many modern popcorn strains. These kernels come in various colors and sizes, offering a wide range of flavors, textures, and visual appeal.

Heirloom popcorn kernels often have more distinctive, nuanced flavors compared to their commercial counterparts. Some examples of heirloom popcorn varieties include Dakota Black, Japanese Hulless, and Strawberry popcorn. By experimenting with heirloom popcorn kernels, you can discover a world of unique popcorn experiences that you won't find at your local movie theater or grocery store.

Debunking the Myth of Hull-less Popcorn Kernels: A Closer Look

As we delve into the diverse world of popcorn kernels, it's crucial to address and debunk a widespread misconception among popcorn enthusiasts: the existence of hull-less popcorn kernels. There are numerous brands that claim that their kernels are "hull-less" and sell them for a more expensive price compared to regular popcorn that we all know and love. In this section, we'll uncover the truth behind the hull-less kernel myth and set the record straight.

The Hull: An Integral Component of the Kernel

First and foremost, it's vital to recognize that all popcorn kernels possess a hull, also known as the pericarp. The hull is the outer shell of the kernel, made up of a tough, fibrous material that encloses the soft endosperm (the starchy part of the kernel that expands when heated and becomes popcorn). The hull is an indispensable part of the kernel, as it supplies the necessary pressure for the kernel to pop when heated. Without a hull, the kernel simply wouldn't be able to turn into popcorn.

The Confusion: Misunderstandings and Misnomers

The confusion surrounding hull-less popcorn kernels arises likely from the fact that some popcorn varieties are marketed as "hull-less" or "virtually hull-less." However, these terms can be deceptive, as they don't actually pertain to kernels without a hull. Instead, these labels are typically used to describe popcorn varieties with a thinner or more delicate hull, which tends to shatter into smaller, less noticeable fragments when the kernel pops.

One such example is the aforementioned ladyfinger popcorn, which has a thin, delicate hull that breaks apart more easily during the popping process. This results in popcorn with fewer noticeable hull fragments, creating a more tender and enjoyable snacking experience. Other popcorn varieties, like some heirloom types, may also have thinner hulls that give a similar result.

The Reality: Seeking a More Tender Popcorn Experience

While it's true that no popcorn kernel is truly hull-less, there are still ways to achieve a more tender and enjoyable popcorn experience. Seeking out popcorn varieties with thinner hulls, such as ladyfinger popcorn or certain heirloom varieties, can help minimize the presence of hull fragments in your popped corn, making for a more pleasant and enjoyable snack.

Additionally, proper storage and preparation of your popcorn kernels can also help reduce the presence of tough or chewy hulls in your popcorn. Keeping your kernels in an airtight container in a cool, dry place will help maintain their moisture content, which is crucial for successful popping. When it comes time to pop your corn, be sure to use high-quality oil and an appropriate heat source to ensure even and thorough popping, which can help reduce the number of un-popped kernels and tough hulls in your finished popcorn.

The realm of popcorn kernels is much more varied and captivating than one might initially think. Ranging from the well-known yellow and white types to the more exotic red, blue, and black kernels, there's a popcorn variety to suit every taste and event. For example, heirloom popcorn kernels bring a rich assortment of distinct flavors and textures to the table, whereas ladyfinger kernels deliver a gentle and refined snacking delight. Even the myth of hull-less popcorn kernels has actually shed light on the significance of hulls and how their varying thicknesses play a key role in the popcorn's overall texture. With a diverse range of options to choose from, delving into the intriguing world of popcorn kernels can truly enhance your snacking adventures. So, when you're organizing your next movie night or just in the mood for a tasty treat, why not experiment with a new variety of popcorn kernels? You might just stumble upon a newfound favorite that has you reaching for more.

Chapter 11

Science of Popping Popcorn

Popcorn is a beloved snack by many due to its many available flavors and nutritional content. Do you ever find yourself mindlessly munching on fluffy, buttery kernels while watching a movie or chatting with friends? Well, have you ever stopped to think about the science behind popcorn's magical transformation from hard kernel to fluffy snack?

It's time to unravel the mystery!

In this chapter, we'll take a deep dive into the captivating science behind popcorn popping. From the anatomy of the kernel to the crucial role of water and heat and even the impact of storage conditions, we'll explore all the elements that make popcorn such a unique and fascinating snack. So, get ready to be amazed and gain a new appreciation for this beloved treat.

Understanding the Popcorn Kernel's Anatomy

To comprehend the reasons behind popcorn's popping action, it's crucial to first familiarize ourselves with the basic structure of a popcorn kernel. Every kernel is made up of three primary components:

The Pericarp: This tough outer shell safeguards the kernel. Mainly composed of cellulose, it's designed to endure a specific amount of pressure.

The Endosperm: This starchy material constitutes most of the kernel's interior. It comprises two kinds of starch molecules: rigid, crystalline starches and soft, amorphous starches.

The Germ: This part of the kernel is the plant's embryo, containing the genetic information necessary for growth. It's enveloped by the endosperm and is located at the kernel's base.

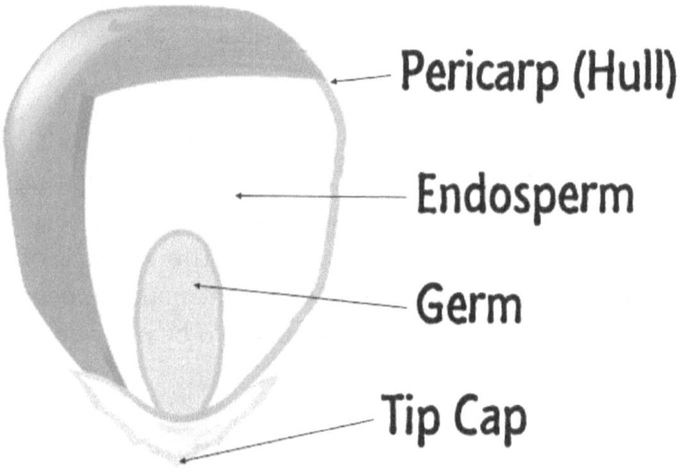

The Role of Water and Heat in the Popping Process

Popcorn's ability to pop is rooted in the interaction between water and heat. Each popcorn kernel holds a small quantity of moisture, roughly 14-20% of its weight. This moisture is vital for the popping process, as it transforms into steam when the kernel is heated. The process unfolds as follows:

As heat is applied to the kernel, the water inside starts to expand and convert into steam.

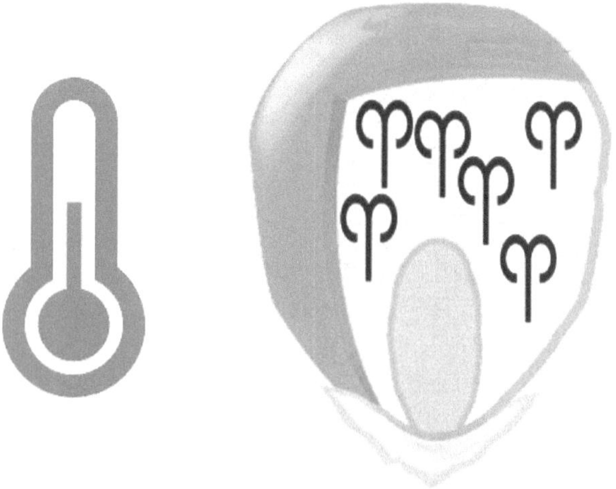

The pressure from the steam builds up within the kernel, causing the temperature inside to rise further.

As the popcorn kernel is heated, the water and oil within it heat up, causing the surrounding starch to soften. The kernel's pericarp, or outer shell, is incredibly tough, preventing the water from escaping when it initially turns into steam. The steam continues to heat up, causing water molecules to move faster and increase the pressure inside the seed.

Eventually, the pericarp can no longer withstand this force and ruptures. In short, the pressure reaches a critical point causing the seed coat to burst open. Upon rupture, the steam rapidly escapes, and the endosperm expands and solidifies, creating the fluffy white popcorn we all know and love.

Upon rupture, the steam rapidly escapes, and the endosperm then expands and solidifies, creating the fluffy white popcorn we all know and love.

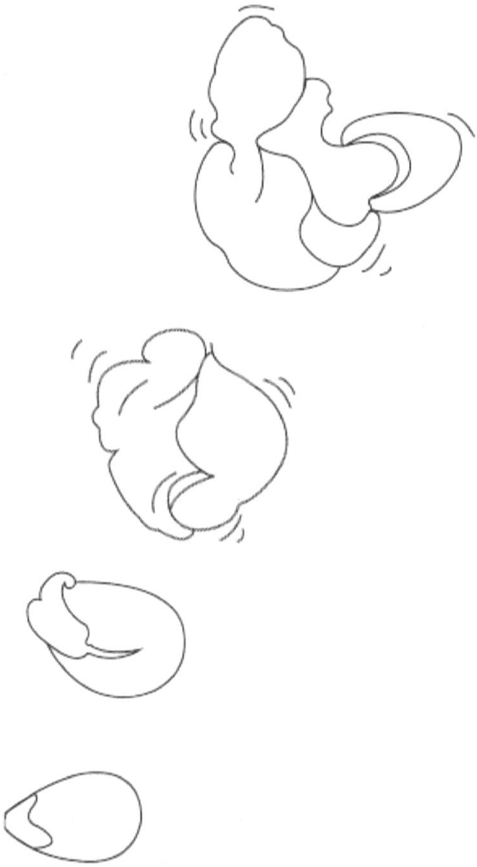

The Crucial Role of the Pericarp in Popping

The pericarp is integral to the popping process, as its strength must be sufficient to endure the internal pressure until the perfect moment. A weak or damaged pericarp may lead to improper popping or failure to pop altogether. Conversely, an overly strong pericarp could necessitate excessive heat and pressure for rupture, resulting in overcooked or scorched popcorn. The pericarp's strength hinges on its structure and composition. It boasts a distinct glassy texture, allowing it to withstand pressure. This characteristic is attributed to a higher concentration of cellulose and lignin, which offer rigidity and durability.

The Uniqueness of Popcorn Among Corn Varieties

Though there are numerous types of corn, only popcorn kernels possess the exceptional blend of qualities that allow them to pop, other types of corn, such as sweet corn, dent corn, and flint corn, have different pericarp structures, and lower moisture content, preventing them from undergoing the popping process. Popcorn belongs to the species Zea mays everta and is distinguished by its rounded, compact kernel shape and the glassy texture of its pericarp. These characteristics allow these kernels to withstand the high pressure and temperature required for popping, whereas other corn varieties would simply dry out or crack under the same conditions.

Popping Methods: From Stovetop to Microwave

The key to perfect popcorn lies in heating the kernels evenly and quickly, allowing the internal pressure to build up and rupture the pericarp at the right moment. Various methods can be used to achieve this, including stovetops, air poppers, and microwaves. Each method has its own advantages and disadvantages:

<u>Stovetop Popping</u>

This traditional method involves heating kernels in a pot with a small amount of oil over medium-high heat. The oil helps to distribute the heat evenly, ensuring that the kernels reach the optimal popping temperature simultaneously. However, it can be challenging to prevent the popcorn from burning, and the oil adds extra calories.

Air Poppers

These electric appliances use hot air to circulate and heat the kernels without the need for oil. This results in a healthier, lower-calorie snack. However, air poppers can sometimes blow un-popped kernels out of the popping chamber, leading to some waste.

Microwave Popping

Microwaves offer a convenient and quick way to make popcorn, using specialized microwave popcorn bags or microwave-safe containers. The microwave's energy causes the water molecules inside the kernels to vibrate and generate heat rapidly, creating the steam pressure necessary for popping. However, microwave popcorn can sometimes be unevenly cooked, and pre-packaged microwave popcorn often contains added fats, salt, and artificial flavors.

The Role of Kernel Shape and Size

Not all popcorn kernels are created equal, and their shape and size can impact their popping performance. Rounder, more symmetrical kernels, such as the mushroom variety, tend to pop more uniformly and produce larger, fluffier popcorn. Smaller, irregularly shaped kernels, like the butterfly kinds, may not heat as evenly, resulting in a higher percentage of un-popped kernels, also known as "old maids" or "spinsters."

The Impact of Storage Conditions

Proper storage is essential for maintaining popcorn's popping ability. As previously mentioned, the moisture content within the kernel is a critical factor in the popping process. If popcorn is stored in a cool, dry place and sealed in an airtight container, it can retain its moisture and remain poppable for an extended period. Conversely, if popcorn is exposed to heat, humidity, or air, it can lose its moisture and become less likely to pop. In some cases, it may be possible to revive stale popcorn by placing it in a sealed container with a small amount of water for a day or two. This allows the kernels to reabsorb some moisture and potentially improve their popping performance.

A Deeper Appreciation for Popcorn

Popcorn is more than just a delicious snack; it's a fascinating display of science at work. Through an understanding of the popcorn kernel's anatomy, the crucial role of water and heat in the popping process, and the importance of factors such as pericarp strength, kernel shape and size, and storage conditions, we can gain a deeper appreciation for this beloved snack. Whether you prefer stovetop popping, air popping, or microwave popping, each method has its advantages and disadvantages, and the perfect batch of popcorn requires attention to detail. So, the next time you enjoy a bowl of popcorn, take a moment to marvel at the complex science that transforms a tiny, hard kernel into a fluffy, delightful treat.

Chapter 12

From Seed to Popcorn

In the heart of America's agricultural epicenter, a remarkable story of transformation unfolds as spring breathes life into the vast expanse of the Corn Belt. Here, amid the fertile fields, farmers embark on a journey that begins with the sowing of seeds – not just any seeds, the foundation of a beloved snack: popcorn. Delicately planted about an inch and a half deep into the soil and spaced with care, these tiny kernels hold the potential to become the fluffy, irresistible bites that captivate our taste buds.

Popcorn Planting

Sowing the Seeds of Promise

As spring unfurls its vibrant tapestry across the Corn Belt, farmers step onto the fields with the seeds of promise in hand. These precious popcorn seeds are planted about an inch and a half deep into the soil, with approximately six inches of space between them. Across an acre of land, nearly 28,000 seeds take root, poised to grow.

The Growth of a Popcorn Plant

Nurtured by Nature

With the seeds now firmly planted in the soil, a remarkable transformation begins. Popcorn seeds respond to the moisture in the earth, which dissolves essential nutrients like nitrogen, phosphate, and potash. The plant's roots act as conduits, absorbing this nutrient-rich moisture to nourish the seed and coax it into germination.

In just a matter of days, the first green shoots emerge, starting the birth of a new popcorn plant. As the sun hits the leaves, a process called photosynthesis unfolds. The chlorophyll within the leaves combines water and carbon dioxide from the air to produce sugar, which fuels the growth of more leaves, roots, and eventually, ears of popcorn.

The popcorn plant reaches its zenith at approximately eight feet in height, its sturdy stalk standing tall and proud. Throughout its growth, the plant requires 18-24 inches of water during the growing season. As it matures, the plant's ears, concealed beneath a protective green husk, begin to form. At the pinnacle of the plant, feathery tassels sway in the wind, releasing golden pollen. Popcorn seeds are planted in clusters to help other plants pollinate the others. Wind plays a part in this process.

Harvest – The Fruit of the Labor!

Nature's Cue

The time for harvest approaches when the popcorn plant stands tall with its stalk and leaves turned brown and dry. A crucial signal, known as the "black layer," appears on the kernels, confirming that the plant is ready. Popcorn is typically harvested when its kernels contain a moisture content of 16%-20%, a vital factor for the ultimate popability.

Harvesting popcorn can be done in two ways. Some opt for ear-harvesting, where the entire ear of corn is carefully cut and then stored for eight to twelve months. During this time, the kernels dry to their ideal moisture levels. Only then are they stripped from the cobs, and any undersized kernels are removed, ensuring that only the cream of the crop remains.

Alternatively, many popcorn farmers turn to the trusty combine for efficient harvesting. This multifunctional machine boasts a "corn head" that efficiently strips the ears from the stalk. The corn is then processed within the combine, separating the kernels from the cob, and ejecting the cob from the rear of the machine. The kernels are loaded onto trucks and transported to storage bins designed with perforated floors, where forced air completes the drying process until the moisture level reaches the optimal 14% – the perfect condition for popping corn.

In some cases, popcorn is harvested on the ear using a corn picker, which deftly removes the entire ear without disturbing the kernels. The corn then dries while still attached to the cob, with the kernels extracted at a later stage.

Processing Popcorn

Polishing Perfection

Once the popcorn kernels have achieved their ideal moisture content of 14%, the meticulous process of cleaning and preparation begins. A series of machines are employed to ensure that every kernel is pristine and ready for its journey to your bowl.

The kernels are first sifted over vibrating screens, which expertly separate them from any lingering cob fragments or other plant materials. Next, they pass through a gravity separator that eliminates lightweight particles, ensuring only robust kernels make the final cut.

Finally, the kernels undergo a polishing process, a meticulous step to eliminate any last remnants of plant material clinging to the kernel's surface. Now, these kernels stand ready to fulfill their destiny, packaged and prepared for microwave bags, glass jars, or bulk distribution. And there you have it, the journey from popcorn's humble beginnings as a tiny seed to the fluffy, irresistible kernels that grace our snack bowls.

So, as you reach for that bowl of popcorn, take a moment to appreciate the journey it has undertaken. From the vibrant fields of the Corn Belt to your snack bowl, it's a story of wonder, nature's marvels, and the human touch that brings it all together. Each kernel is a bite-sized testament to the rich bounty of the Corn Belt and the enchanting world of popcorn. Enjoy the show!

Chapter 13

The Best Oil to Pop Popcorn

Popcorn has long been a cherished snack enjoyed by countless people around the world, be it at movie theaters or in the cozy environment of our own homes. Have you ever given thought to the best oil for popping those delightful, fluffy kernels? In this chapter, we invite you to join us on a delectable journey as we delve into the various oils that are ideal for making popcorn. Uncover how distinct oils can enhance the flavors and textures of your go-to treat and find out why selecting the right oil is essential for the ultimate popcorn indulgence.

Coconut Oil

Its high smoke point (about 350°F, or 177°C) renders it well-suited for high-temperature cooking methods like popcorn making. It's worth mentioning that there are also different types of this oil. Unrefined coconut oil boasts a pronounced coconut taste that may not pair well with unflavored popcorn. Refined coconut oil, on the other hand, has a milder flavor and a higher smoke point, making it a more suitable choice. Additionally, coconut oil is abundant in medium-chain triglycerides (MCTs) that are easily absorbed and metabolized into energy by the body. This characteristic places it ahead of oils high in saturated fats in terms of health benefits. However, use this in moderation as it can have high-calorie content.

When we pop popcorn without a candy coating, typically our butter or seasoned flavors, we use a butter coconut oil which adds just a little extra flavor when popping.

Corn Oil

Corn oil is a popular choice for popping popcorn because of its high smoke point and mild flavor.

Corn oil's smoke point is typically around 450°F (232°C). This means it can handle the high temperatures required for popping popcorn without breaking down and producing a burnt taste or harmful smoke.

We like corn oil because of its neutral, mild flavor. This neutrality allows the natural taste of the popcorn to shine through which is why this is our go to oil for popping corn with coatings such as kettle corn, caramel corn, and other candy-coated flavorings. Corn oil won't overpower the popcorn's inherent flavor.

It is relatively low in saturated fats and contains a good amount of polyunsaturated fats, primarily omega-6 fatty acids.

Canola Oil

Canola oil offers another popular alternative for popcorn preparation. Its high smoke point of approximately 400°F (204°C) enables it to withstand the heat necessary to pop the kernels without generating harmful smoke. Furthermore, canola oil's low saturated fat content and high monounsaturated fat content make it a heart-friendly option. A notable advantage of using canola oil is its neutral taste, which highlights the popcorn's inherent flavor. This attribute makes it a flexible choice for those eager to try various seasoning combinations without overwhelming the popcorn's taste.

Olive Oil

For a more adventurous take on your popcorn, consider olive oil. This Mediterranean staple is praised for its health benefits, owing to its high concentration of monounsaturated fats and antioxidants. To maximize both flavor and nutrition, opt for extra virgin olive oil. While olive oil's smoke point (about 320°F or 160°C) is lower compared to other oils on this list, it can still be employed for making popcorn as long as you carefully monitor the temperature. The oil imparts a rich, fruity undertone to the popcorn, resulting in a delectable and distinctive snack. To infuse a Mediterranean flair, try seasoning your olive oil-popped popcorn with herbs such as rosemary, thyme, or oregano.

Sunflower Oil

Sunflower oil is a great choice for popcorn making, thanks to its high smoke point (around 450°F, or 232°C) and mild flavor. It's also high in vitamin E, an antioxidant that helps protect cells from damage and supports a healthy immune system. Sunflower oil is low in saturated fats and high in polyunsaturated fats, making it a heart-healthy choice. Its neutral taste makes it a versatile option for various popcorn flavorings, from sweet to savory. For an extra nutritious twist, look for high-oleic sunflower oil, which is even higher in monounsaturated fats.

Avocado Oil

Avocado oil is a newer addition to the popcorn-popping scene, but it's quickly gaining popularity for its high smoke point (520°F or 271°C) and exceptional health benefits. Rich in monounsaturated fats and antioxidants, avocado oil supports heart health and has anti-inflammatory properties. The oil has a buttery, slightly nutty flavor that adds depth to your popcorn, making it a delicious and nutritious choice. Its high smoke point ensures that the oil won't break down during the popping process, preserving its nutritional qualities. Avocado oil's versatility also makes it suitable for various popcorn seasonings, from spicy to sweet.

Ghee

Ghee, a form of clarified butter, is a popular choice among popcorn connoisseurs for its rich, buttery flavor. It is made by simmering butter to remove the water content and milk solids, resulting in a golden, flavorful fat that imparts a delicious buttery taste to your popcorn. While ghee is high in saturated fat, it also contains short-chain fatty acids and conjugated linoleic acid (CLA), which have been linked to various health benefits, such as supporting digestion and a healthy immune system. However, moderation is still key when using ghee, especially for those watching their fat intake.

Peanut Oil

Peanut oil is another excellent choice for popping popcorn, offering a unique, nutty flavor. Its mild taste allows the popcorn's natural flavors to shine through while adding a hint of nuttiness that many find irresistible. Peanut oil is high in monounsaturated fats, which support heart health, and it's also a good source of vitamin E. However, be cautious when serving peanut oil-popped popcorn to guests, as some individuals may have peanut allergies.

Oil Tips for Popcorn Popping

Now that you know the best types of oils for popping popcorn, keep these tips in mind to ensure a perfect batch every time:

Use the right amount of oil. A good ratio of oil to popcorn is key. It depends on the type of popcorn popper you are using which dictates the right ratio of oil to kernels. Typically, an auto stirring popper would use the following ratios to pop great popcorn.

Popper Size	Oil	Kernels
4oz	1oz	4oz
6oz	2oz	6oz
8oz	3oz	8oz
12/14oz	4oz	12 or 14oz
16oz	5oz	16oz
20oz	6oz	20oz

If you are using a large kettle and hand stirring, you may want to change the ratio slightly. We prefer to use half the amount of oil as we do kernels in order to allow for easier and smoother stirring.

Preheat the oil: Before adding the kernels, heat the oil. Wait for it to shimmer before adding the popcorn – this will ensure that the kernels heat up quickly and pop evenly. If you are popping in a theater style popcorn popper or kettle it's okay to add the oil and kernels at the same time as long as you've heated the kettle first.

Keep it moving: As the popcorn pops, it's important to keep the kernels moving to distribute the heat and prevent the kernels from sticking or burning.

Allow steam to escape when possible so your popcorn stays crisp and doesn't become soggy.

Season immediately: Add your choice of seasoning as soon as the popcorn is done popping while it's still hot and coated in oil to ensure the flavors stick.

The best types of oil for popping popcorn are those with high smoke points and complementary flavors. Coconut oil, corn oil, canola oil, olive oil, sunflower oil, avocado oil, ghee, and peanut oil are all excellent choices, each offering its unique taste and health benefits. By experimenting with different oils and seasonings, you can create a wide variety of popcorn flavors to suit any craving. So go ahead, grab your favorite oil, and start popping – it's time to enjoy the ultimate popcorn experience!

Chapter 14

How to Pop Popcorn

Popcorn, a beloved snack enjoyed by millions worldwide, has various popping methods at our disposal; each one offers a unique approach to creating the perfect batch of popcorn. From the convenience of microwave popcorn to the traditional stovetop method, the delightful crunch of air-popped popcorn, or the irresistible taste of theater-style popcorn, there's a method to suit every preference and occasion. As we explore the different ways to pop popcorn, let's dive into the techniques, advantages, and nuances of each method and discover the secrets to making the ultimate popcorn experience.

Microwave Popcorn: A Convenient and Tasty Snacking Option

The magic of microwave popcorn lies in its ability to transform kernels into puffy, flavorful snacks within minutes. The process relies on the microwave's electromagnetic waves, which agitate the water molecules within the kernels. As the water heats and turns into steam, the pressure inside the kernel builds. Eventually, the kernel's shell gives way, and the starchy interior explodes into the fluffy, irregular shape we all know and love.

Packaged Popcorn Bags

Microwave popcorn bags are pre-packaged with the perfect combination of kernels, oil, and flavorings. These bags are lined with a susceptor, a thin layer of metal that absorbs microwave energy and converts it into heat. This heat is then evenly distributed across the kernels, causing them to pop.

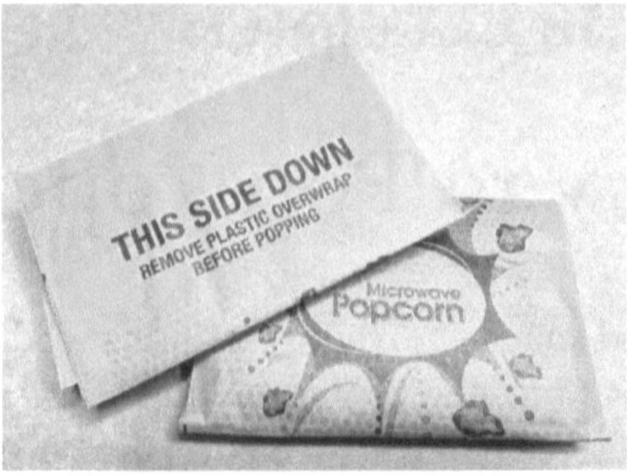

Microwave Popcorn Bags

Weighing the Pros and Cons

What makes microwave popcorn a favorite of many is that it is incredibly convenient, only requiring a few minutes and little effort to prepare. It also allows for a wide variety of flavors, from classic butter and salt to more adventurous options like caramel, cheese, and jalapeño. However, one of its significant drawbacks is its reliance on artificial additives and preservatives, which may not be as healthy as popcorn popped using other methods. Additionally, microwave popcorn bags can sometimes lead to uneven popping or burnt popcorn due to varying microwave power levels and cooking times.

Tips for Microwave Popcorn

To make the most of your microwave popcorn experience, consider these tips:

- Read the instructions: Different brands and flavors may require specific cooking times, so always consult the packaging for the best results.
- Listen closely: When the popping slows down to about 2-3 seconds between pops, it's time to stop the microwave. Overcooking may result in burnt popcorn.

- Shake it up: Gently shake the bag before and after microwaving to distribute the oil and seasonings evenly and prevent the kernels from sticking together. Hold the bag from the bottom and shake it over a garbage pail upside down. This will allow any un-popped kernels to come out.
- Vent the bag: After removing the bag from the microwave, let it sit for a moment to allow steam to escape. This prevents the popcorn from getting soggy.
- Get creative: if you're craving a unique flavor, try adding your favorite seasonings, such as nutritional yeast, garlic powder, or chili powder, to customize your popcorn experience.

By following these tips and experimenting with flavors, you can enjoy delicious and convenient microwave popcorn whenever the craving strikes.

Stovetop Popcorn: The Classic Method for Popping Perfection

There are two stovetop methods you can use.

Oil-Based Method

The oil-based method is the most common technique for stovetop popcorn popping. With this approach, you'll need a large pot with a lid, your preferred cooking oil, and popcorn kernels. Heat the oil in the pot, add the kernels, and then cover the pot with a lid. As the kernels heat up, they'll start to pop. Continuously shake the pot to ensure even cooking and prevent burning. Once the popping slows down, remove the pot from the heat and let it rest for a moment before unveiling your delicious, homemade popcorn.

Dry Popping

Dry popping, also known as "dry roasting," is a less common but equally delicious method for stovetop popcorn making. This technique requires no oil, making it a healthier option for those looking to cut back on calories. To dry pop, place the kernels in a large pot with a lid, and heat them over medium heat. Shake the pot frequently to prevent burning and ensure even cooking. Once the popping subsides, remove the pot from the heat and enjoy your oil-free stovetop popcorn.

Advantages and Disadvantages

Popping popcorn on the stovetop allows you to customize the ingredients and taste, letting you create a snack that's just right for your preferences. You can enjoy trying out various oils, seasonings, and toppings, whether you opt for oil-based or dry-popping methods. However, stovetop popcorn does demand more care compared to microwave popcorn. You'll need to watch the heat and shake the pot occasionally. Also, there's a higher risk of scorching the popcorn if you're not careful.

Tips for Stovetop Popcorn

Follow these tips to master the art of stovetop popcorn popping:

- Choose the right pot: Opt for a heavy-bottomed pot with a tight-fitting lid to ensure even heat distribution and prevent burning.
- Preheat the oil: If using the oil-based method, make sure to preheat the oil before adding the kernels. To test if the oil is hot enough, add a single kernel; if it spins or pops, the oil is ready.
- Don't layer the kernels: Spread the kernels in a single layer on the bottom of the pot for even cooking.
- Shake, shake, shake: Keep the pot moving to prevent the popcorn from sticking and burning.
- Season to taste: Get creative with your seasonings – try a sprinkle of sea salt, a dash of nutritional yeast, or a hint of smoked paprika for a unique flavor experience.

By mastering the stovetop popcorn method, you'll enjoy a delicious, homemade snack that's perfect for movie nights, gatherings, or whenever you're craving a crunchy, satisfying treat.

Theater Style Popcorn: Elevates the Cinema Experience

Commercial popcorn machines, like the ones found in movie theaters, use a combination of heat and agitation to pop kernels uniformly and efficiently. These machines typically feature a heated kettle with a built-in stirring mechanism, ensuring the kernels are evenly coated with oil and preventing them from sticking together or burning. Once the popcorn is popped, it's funneled into a heated compartment, which keeps it warm and crisp until it's ready to be served.

<u>The Key Components of Theater-Style Popcorn</u>

Oil

The oil used in theater-style popcorn plays a significant role in its distinct taste and texture. Many commercial popcorn machines use coconut oil, which has a high smoke point and imparts a subtle, sweet flavor. This oil not only contributes to the popcorn's overall taste but also helps create that signature golden color.

Seasoning

Theater-style popcorn is incomplete without its signature seasoning. The most common seasoning used in movie theaters is Flavacol, a fine, butter-flavored salt that dissolves quickly and evenly coats the popcorn. Flavacol's vibrant yellow color also adds to the visual appeal of theater-style popcorn.

Flavacol Quantities for Popping Butter Popcorn

Popper Size	Oil	Flavacol
4oz	1oz	1 tsp
6oz	2oz	1/2 TBS
8oz	3oz	1 TBS
12/14oz	4oz	1 1/2 TBS
16oz	5oz	1 1/2 TBS
20oz	6oz	2 TBS
32oz to 36oz	9.5oz	3 TBS
48oz to 52oz	15oz	5 TBS
60oz	18oz	6 TBS

Advantages and Disadvantages

Theater-style popcorn's irresistible taste and aroma are its biggest selling points. The combination of oil and seasoning creates a delicious, crave-worthy snack that's hard to resist. Additionally, commercial popcorn machines can produce large quantities of popcorn quickly, making them ideal for gatherings or events. One of the disadvantages of theater-style popcorn is its calorie count. The oil and seasoning used can significantly increase the snack's fat and sodium content. Additionally, commercial popcorn machines can be expensive and may require regular maintenance.

Theater-style popcorn provides a nostalgic and flavorful snacking experience that's hard to beat. While it may not be the healthiest option, it's certainly a treat worth indulging in from time to time. If you're looking to recreate this cinema classic at home, consider investing in a smaller countertop popcorn machine and experimenting with different oils and seasonings to find the perfect combination for your taste buds.

Air Popper: A Healthier Way to Enjoy Popcorn

Air poppers work using two key elements to pop kernels without the need for oil or gas: the principle of hot air circulation and the actual circulation process.

The Role of Hot Air Circulation

Air poppers have become a favorite among health-minded popcorn lovers since they rely on hot air instead of oil to pop the kernels. These machines come with a heating element that quickly heats up the air within the popper. As the air becomes hot, it circulates around the kernels, causing them to heat up and eventually pop.

Popping Chamber

The popping chamber in an air popper is specifically designed to facilitate even heat distribution and ensure that all kernels are exposed to hot air. Once the kernels pop, they are expelled from the chamber and into a waiting bowl, providing a quick, mess-free popcorn experience.

Advantages and Disadvantages

Air poppers present a healthier choice compared to conventional oil-popped popcorn since they skip the added fats. This leads to a lower calorie treat that's equally delightful. Additionally, air poppers are user-friendly and a breeze to clean, making them a practical choice for on-the-go families. One downside of air-popped popcorn is that it can sometimes be less flavorful than its oil-popped counterparts, as the lack of oil makes it harder for seasonings to adhere to the popcorn. Additionally, air poppers may not always produce popped kernels evenly, resulting in a mix of fully popped and partially popped pieces.

Tips for Better Air-Popped Popcorn

To enhance your air-popped popcorn experience, consider these tips:

- Season immediately: Add seasonings to the popcorn as soon as it's expelled from the popper to help the flavor stick better.
- Get creative with toppings: Experiment with various healthy toppings like nutritional yeast, cinnamon, or chili powder to add flavor without adding excessive calories.
- Store kernels properly: Keep your popcorn kernels in an airtight container to maintain their freshness and ensure optimal popping results.

By following these tips and embracing the simplicity of air poppers, you can enjoy a healthier and more delicious popcorn snack anytime the craving strikes.

Hand Crank: A Fun and Flavorful Stovetop Popcorn Experience

The hand cranked stovetop popper offers a one-of-a-kind popcorn-making experience by blending the best features of classic stovetop and commercial popcorn machines. This lightweight aluminum pan comes with an integrated stirring mechanism controlled by a crank on the popper's exterior. Hand cranked popcorn poppers are designed to release steam, making sure your popcorn stays crunchy and fresh while cooking.

Popping Process

A hand cranked popper simplifies the stovetop popping process by providing even heat distribution and constant stirring, which prevents the kernels from sticking or burning. To use a hand cranked popper, add your desired oil and popcorn kernels to the pan, place it on the stovetop, and begin turning the crank. As the kernels heat and begin to pop, the stirring mechanism ensures that they are evenly coated in oil and cook uniformly.

Advantages and Disadvantages

A hand cranked popper offers several advantages over the traditional stovetop method, including more control over the ingredients, faster cooking times, and a higher yield of fully popped kernels. The built-in stirring mechanism also allows for easy experimentation with different flavors and seasonings, resulting in a personalized popcorn experience. One potential drawback of a hand cranked popper is the need for a stovetop and manual stirring, which may be less convenient than a microwave or electric popcorn machines. Additionally, the aluminum construction may be less durable than other heavy-duty stovetop pots.

To ensure deliciously, perfectly popped hand cranked popcorn, follow these tips:

- Preheat the popper: Warm the popper over medium heat before adding the oil and kernels to promote even cooking.
- Use high-quality ingredients: Choose quality popcorn kernels and oil for the best flavor and texture.
- Experiment with flavors: Get creative with seasonings and toppings to create your ideal popcorn snack.

By mastering hand cranked popcorn popper, you'll enjoy a fun and interactive popcorn-making experience that results in a delicious, homemade snack perfect for movie nights, parties, or simply satisfying your popcorn cravings.

Kettle Corn Machine

A Kettle Corn Machine is an apparatus that creates sweet and savory popcorn delights. Crafted with precision and purpose, this specialized popcorn popper is dedicated solely to the art of crafting the perfect batch of kettle corn.

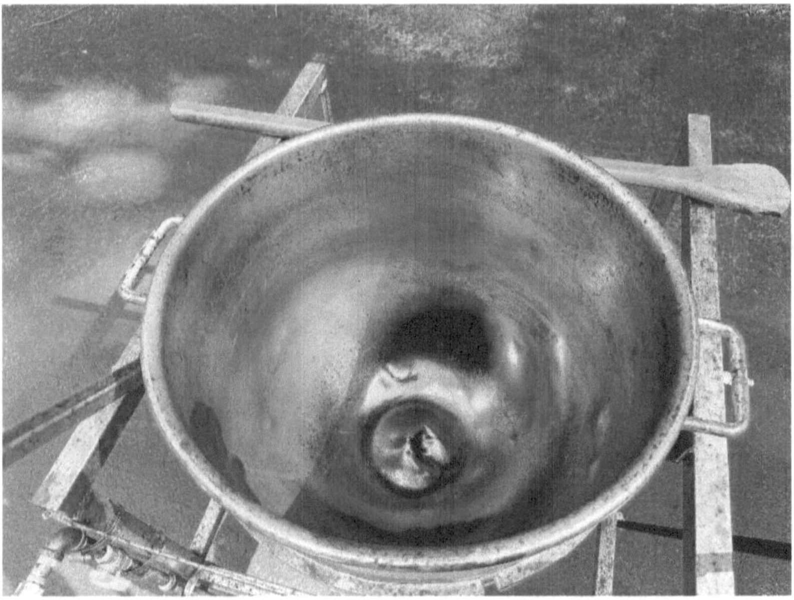

Kettle Corn Machine

At its core, the Kettle Corn Machine features a spacious kettle adorned with a heating element and a stirring mechanism. The stirring mechanism can be automatic, but it can also be stirred manually. Typically that involves a person with a big wooden paddle stirring the kernels and popcorn. Its size varies, from the intimate 60-quart model to the grandeur of 180 quarts, each meticulously crafted from materials such as stainless steel, cast iron, or the elegant allure of copper.

The process of popping kettle corn is not extremely difficult in fact here is a run-down of how kettle corn is typically made.

1. Preparation: Begin by meticulously measuring out the required quantities of oil and popcorn kernels. The amount you will use depends on the size of the kettle, but using the appropriate ratio is necessary. You will want to use half the amount of oil that you have for kernels. So if you are using 3 cups of kernels, you will use 1 ½ cups of oil. You will also want to get your sugar ready. Typically you will use the same amount of sugar as you are oil. So in our example, you will use 1 ½ cups of sugar.
2. Ignition: Activate the burner either by flicking a switch, lighting it with a lighter, or igniting it with a match. The flames will start initiating the heating process necessary for popcorn perfection.

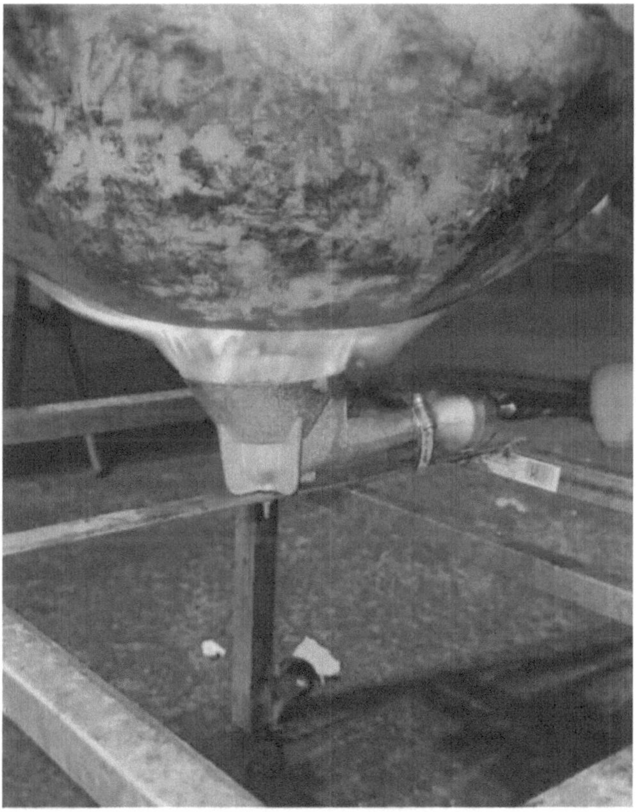

Lighting Kettle Corn Machine Burner

3. Ingredients: Add the oil and kernels to the kettle and allow it to heat up.

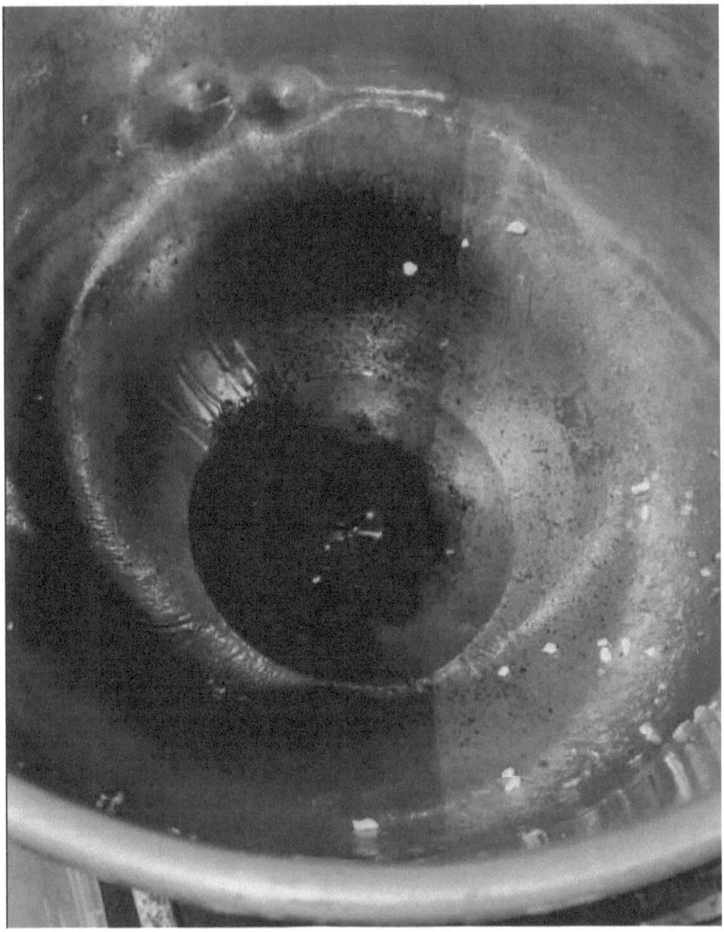

Oil in Kettle Corn Machine

4. Stirring: As the kettle warms, engage the stirring mechanism to agitate the kernels evenly or begin mixing by hand with a paddle. This crucial step prevents uneven heating and ensures every kernel receives its fair share of heat.

5. Popping: With the rising temperature, the kernels begin to pop. Once they start it's time to add in the sugar. You will continue to stir the popcorn for even heating and to prevent burning.

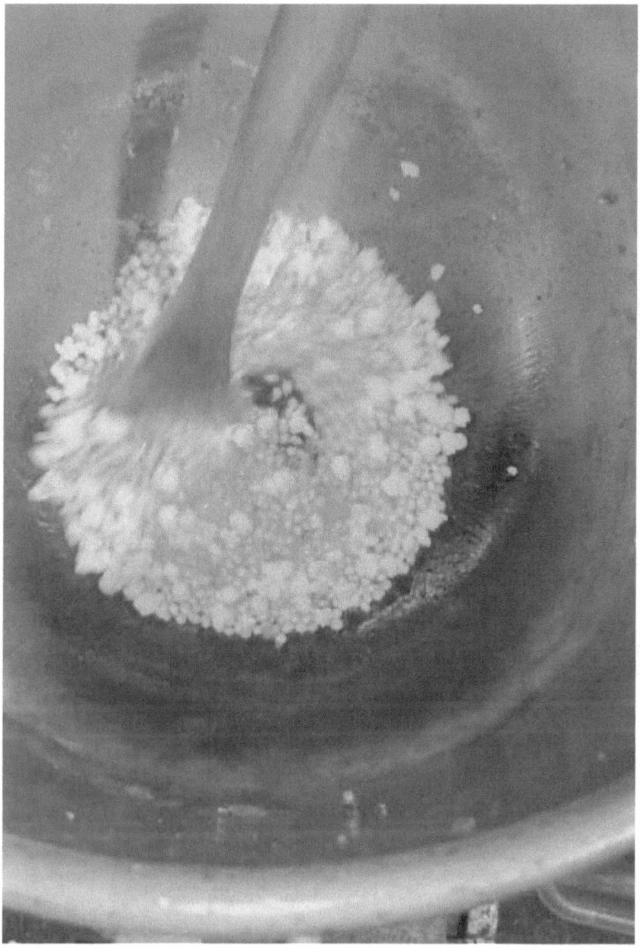

Kernels Popping

6. Culmination: As the popping diminishes, the kettle unveils perfectly popped kettle corn with the perfect balance of sweetness.

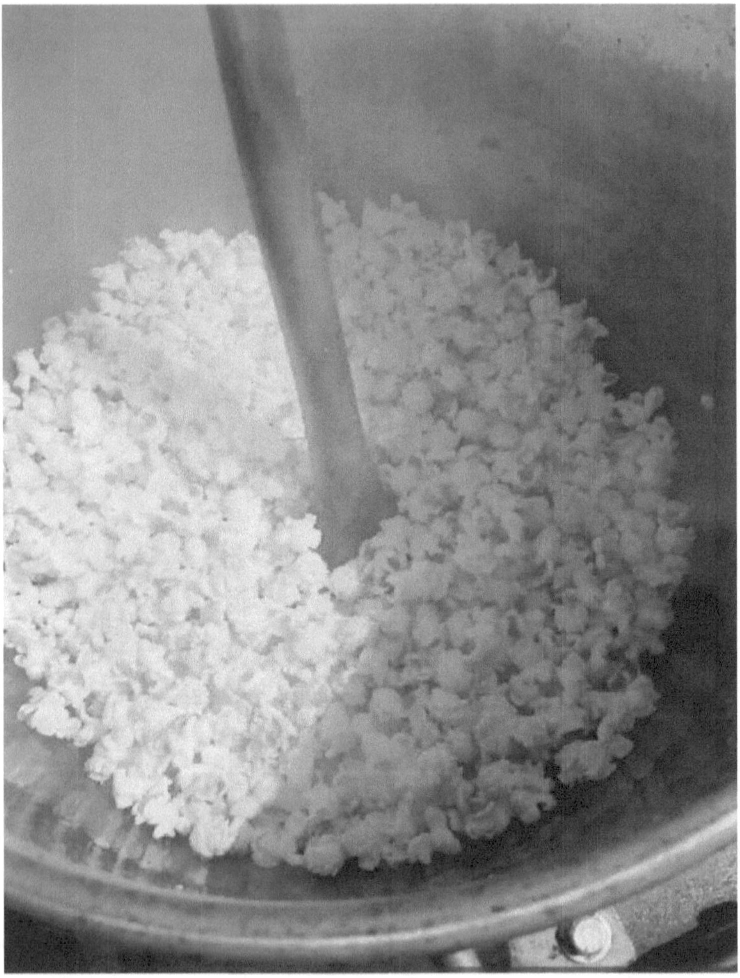

Popped Kettle Corn

7. Seasoning: Complete the transformation by sprinkling a dash of salt over the freshly popped kettle corn.

And thus, from the depths of the Kettle Corn Machine emerges a delicious popcorn taste. Sweet and savory, crisp and golden, it is a delight to be savored and shared.

Unique and Intriguing Ways to Pop Popcorn

Popcorn is a versatile snack that can be popped using a variety of methods. In addition to the traditional techniques we've already discussed, there are several unconventional and unique ways to prepare popcorn that you might not have considered. Let's explore some of these lesser-known methods that offer a fun and interesting twist on this beloved snack.

Campfire Popcorn

Campfire popcorn is an easy and entertaining way to enjoy a snack while camping or relaxing around a fire pit. Simply place popcorn kernels in a fire-safe container or heavy-duty aluminum foil pouch and suspend it over the campfire. As the kernels heat, they'll absorb a delicious smoky flavor, making for a tasty and memorable outdoor treat.

Grilled Popcorn

During warm summer months, the grill becomes a popular spot for cooking all sorts of dishes. To make grilled popcorn, place kernels in a grill-safe container or wrap them in heavy-duty aluminum foil, then place the package on the grill. As the kernels pop, they'll take on a subtly smoky flavor, creating a unique and delicious snack that's perfect for backyard barbecues.

Wok Popcorn

Using a wok to pop popcorn may not be as unconventional as other methods, but it does offer a unique and even heat distribution, which results in perfectly popped kernels. To make wok popcorn, heat a small amount of oil in a large wok with a lid, then add popcorn kernels. Continuously stir or toss the kernels to ensure even cooking and avoid burning. The result is a delicious, evenly popped snack with a delightful crunch.

Jiffy Pop

Jiffy Pop is a pre-packaged stovetop popcorn product that became popular in the 1950s. The disposable aluminum pan contains popcorn kernels and oil, which are heated on a stovetop or campfire. As the kernels pop, the expanding aluminum foil cover creates a fun, visually appealing experience. Though Jiffy Pop may not be as widely used today, it remains a nostalgic and convenient option for a quick and easy popcorn snack.

Heat Gun Popcorn

A heat gun may not be the most practical popcorn-popping method, but it demonstrates the versatility of this beloved snack. By directing the heat gun's hot air onto a container of popcorn kernels, you can achieve a unique and entertaining popcorn experience.

Popping Popcorn on the Cob

Contrary to popular belief, popcorn kernels can be popped while still on the cob. Simply wrap a dried popcorn corn cob in heavy-duty aluminum foil, leaving some room for expansion, and place it on a heat source like a stovetop or grill. As the kernels heat and pop, they'll transform the cob into a beautiful and delicious snack, showcasing the natural origins of this versatile treat.

Fried Popcorn

Fried popcorn offers a decadent twist on the classic snack. By frying popcorn kernels in hot oil, they quickly pop and become infused with a rich, buttery flavor. This method results in a crispy texture and intense flavor that doesn't become soggy like some other buttered popcorn options. Experiment with different oils or seasonings to create a truly unique and indulgent popcorn experience.

We've explored various popcorn-popping methods, each with its own unique advantages and characteristics. From the convenience of microwave popcorn to the classic appeal of stovetop popping, the interactive experience of a hand cranked popper to the healthier alternative offered by air poppers, there truly is a method for every preference and occasion. Moreover, we've discovered that innovation and creativity abound in the world of popcorn, with unconventional methods like campfire popcorn, grilled popcorn, and even heat gun popcorn proving that the sky's the limit when it comes to this versatile snack.

Chapter 15

Recipes and Techniques

You've learned a lot about popcorn throughout this book, but one of the best things about popcorn is eating it. This is why we are including some of our personal recipes and techniques for popping gourmet flavored popcorn.

We make our flavored popcorn using the mushroom variety of popcorn. We like this variety because it pops up larger than others and it's very hearty. What we mean by hearty is that it holds up really well when we coat it in candy coatings as well as it doesn't tend to break apart as much when stirring.

We typically make flavored popcorn using one of three different machines. We either use a big kettle, a theater style popcorn popper, or a carmelizer. In this chapter we are also going to include recipes for making popcorn on the stove using a hand crank style popper as not everyone has larger machines. You don't need big machinery to make wonderfully flavored popcorn, you just need an imagination, and some know how.

Our instructions and recipes in this chapter are for specific quantities, but you can pop corn in any quantities, just keep in mind the main ratios that we are using, and you should be perfectly fine in using any quantities based on the size machines that you have.

We are going to categorize our flavor creation process into four basic categories, savory, butter, kettle, and other sweet flavors. Savory flavors include items such as ranch, sriracha, ghost pepper, bacon, cheese, BBQ, etc. You can repeat our strategies with many different flavors by keeping these processes in mind.

For savory flavors, we pop popcorn in butter coconut oil and then after it's fully popped and hot, we sprinkle seasonings on top, coat the popcorn in the seasoning by either shaking the popcorn and seasoning it in a food safe bag or mixing the popcorn and seasoning around in a container. There are also machines that can help you do this as well, but we've always done in by hand.

For butter flavor, we pop popcorn in butter coconut oil and add Flavacol during the popping process. After it finishes popping you have a movie theater salty butter flavored popcorn. People love this simple flavor and we do too.

For kettle corn, we pop popcorn in corn oil and add sugar right when it starts to pop. Once it's fully popped, we add salt to taste so you get that wonderful sweet and savory flavor. For other sweet flavors, such as caramel, chocolate, toffee, grape, lemon, blue raspberry, apple, etc., we make them in one of two ways, we either use the kettle corn technique by adding flavored sugar as the popcorn begins to pop in corn oil, or we pop popcorn in butter coconut oil, let it cool, and then add a candy coating to it afterwards using a carmelizer or copper kettle. After the final step of making sugar coated popcorn it's important to mix it around to cool it using popcorn scoops.

A sifter can come in handy as well as once the popcorn is finished a sifter can help you remove the un-popped kernels from the batch of popcorn.

Aside from the techniques we are outlining in this chapter, we like to coat and drizzle flavored popcorn with melted chocolate along with adding other candies, toppings, and cereals. This makes the number of varieties of flavored popcorn you can make infinite.

<u>The Machines</u>

Now that you understand the different flavoring processes we use, let's talk about the different machines we use to make flavored popcorn.

The Kettle

We pop larger batches of popcorn in a kettle popper. This is the style popper you would typically see at fairs and farmers markets. Our kettle is 60 quarts in size, and we made it ourselves using a dough bowl from a big mixer. We will spare you the details on the construction, but we basically taught ourselves to weld and created our own kettle popper. We even created plans to help others build a similar machine and folks from all over the world have used them to make their own. Enough about that, let's talk about how we make corn in it.

The first thing we do is start heating up the kettle. We start the gas and use a long lighter to ignite it. Once it's lit, we add the kernels and oil. We prefer to use a long wooden paddle and we stir the ingredients around to keep them in motion. During the popping process, the kernels will start to pop and will increase in frequency until almost all the kernels are completely popped. While this is happening, we continue to stir the mixture. When popping slows down, we turn off the heat and dump out the popcorn into a container.

Our 60-quart kettle can handle 3 cups of un-popped kernels very easily. We use a ratio of 2:1 kernels to oil. This allows us to easily hand stir the kernels and popcorn during the popping process. So, in our case we use 3 cups of un-popped kernels to 1 ½ cups of oil. Depending on the size kettle you have, you may use more or less, but if you keep this ratio in mind, you should be good to go.

Let's talk about the different popping processes we use with the kettle:

Savory Flavors

We pop 3 cups of kernels and 1 ½ cups of butter coconut oil. Once the popcorn finishes popping but while it's still hot, we add 2/3 cup of popcorn seasoning and either shake it all together in a food safe bag to coat it or stir it around in a container. We find that adding the seasoning while the kernels are still hot allows it to coat better.

Butter Popcorn

We add 3 cups of kernels, 1 ½ cups of butter coconut oil and 2 TBSP of Flavacol to the kettle and continue stirring until the popcorn pops completely. At the end you have nice buttery flavored popcorn.

Kettle Corn

When we make sweet and savory kettle corn in our machine, we use a 2:1 ratio of kernels to sugar and kernels to oil, which means 3 cups of kernels to 1 ½ cups of sugar. Again, you can repeat this in other machines, just keep the ratio in mind. To make this we add 1 ½ cups of corn oil to the kettle along with 3 cups of corn. When the popcorn begins popping, we add in 1 ½ cups of sugar. One thing you'll notice when you add sugar is that the popping will stop temporarily. This is perfectly normal and is due to adding sugar that is at a lower temperature than the oil, kernel mixture. The mixture now has to come back up to temperature for the kernels to begin popping again. You must continue to stir this throughout the entire process to keep the mixture from burning. Once the popping slows, turn off heat and move kernels to another container, salt it to taste.

Other Sweet Flavors

When we make other sweet flavors in the kettle we use a similar process as we do with making kettle corn except we utilize flavored sugars. We get these flavored sugars by either making our own with extracts or we purchase already made flavored sugars or Glaze Pop. Glaze Pop is a product made by Gold Medal Products and makes very nice, flavored popcorn. The recipes in this chapter will provide some specifics around those other flavored sugars we purchase. To make these we use a 2:1 ratio of kernels to flavored sugar and kernels to oil. In our case, 3 cups of kernels, 1 ½ cups oil, and 1 ½ cups of sugar.

We use corn oil when making sweet flavors in the kettle. To make these, you will use the same technique you do when making kettle corn, but instead of plan sugar you will use the flavored sugar. We also don't add salt to our sweet flavors at the end but some people do. It's really a matter of preference.

The kettle popper serves as the cornerstone of our popcorn-making process, evoking the charm of fairs and farmers markets. With its capacity and a well-maintained ratio of kernels to oil, it provides the perfect canvas for popcorn perfection. From savory to sweet, a kettle corn machine is a very versatile device which can allow you to make an infinite number of flavor combinations.

The Theater Style Popper

We pop popcorn in our theater style popper when we are looking to make smaller batches. Lately we've been using a 6oz theater style popper which means it holds 6oz of un-popped kernels. When we had our popcorn shop in operation, we used our 20oz theater style popcorn popper. For the purpose of this book we are going to explain everything using quantities for our 6oz popper, but again, you can use these techniques with any size just utilize the same ratios. What you'll notice with using a theater style popcorn popper is that you can get a way with using less oil, because of the automatic stirring mechanism. This mechanism allows for a few really great things, less oil means healthier popcorn and cheaper to make. Also, it's less work in having to continue to stir the mixture over and over for the life of the batch.

The basic technique for using a theater style popcorn popper is to start heating the kettle which is usually done by flipping a switch. Depending on the model this can take 5 to 10 minutes. After it's heated, you turn on the motor which is what powers the stirring mechanism. Add your oil and kernels and pop it until the popping sound begins to slow. At that point, you dump out the kettle. Afterwards you turn off the heat and motor. We will get into more specifics in each section below.

This is a great chart that shows the kernels to oil ratios you can use for a theater style popper that is equipped with an automatic stirring mechanism:

Popper Size	Oil	Kernels
4oz	1oz	4oz
6oz	2oz	6oz
8oz	3oz	8oz
12/14oz	4oz	12 or 14oz
16oz	5oz	16oz
20oz	6oz	20oz

Popping Processes using the Theater Popper

Savory Flavors

As we mentioned, our popper is a 6oz size, so we use 6oz of popcorn kernels and 2oz of butter coconut oil. We heat up the kettle and then start the motor once it gets up to temperature. We then add the oil and popcorn kernels and allow the machine to do the work of popping the popcorn. Once the popping slows, we dump the kettle. While the popcorn is still hot, we add ¼ cup of popcorn seasoning. You can either stir the seasoning in to mix it or toss it inside a food safe bag.

Butter Popcorn

For butter flavor, we heat up the kettle, turn on the stirring mechanism and add 6oz of kernels, 2oz of butter coconut oil, and 1 tsp of Flavacol. You can add more Flavacol, but this is a matter of your personal preference. We continue to pop the corn until popping slows down and then dump the kettle. This makes a great movie theater butter flavored popcorn.

This chart shows ratios on how much Flavacol to use based on the size popper that you have.

Popper Size	Oil	Flavacol
4oz	1oz	1 tsp
6oz	2oz	1/2 TBS
8oz	3oz	1 TBS
12/14oz	4oz	1 ½ TBS
16oz	5oz	1 1/2 TBS
20oz	6oz	2 TBS
32oz to 36oz	9.5oz	3 TBS
48oz to 52oz	15oz	5 TBS
60oz	18oz	6 TBS

Kettle Corn

We get asked frequently if it's possible to make kettle corn in a theater style popper and the answer is an astounding yes! To make kettle corn, the basic premise is the same. We heat up the kettle, and once it comes to temperature, we turn on the motor and add 6oz of kernels along with 2oz of corn oil, once it begins popping, we open the lid and add 3oz of sugar. We close the lid, and the popping will start again after the mixture gets back up to temperature. The popping will increase in frequency and crescendo. Once the popping begins to slow down, we dump the kettle and shake on some salt to taste.

Other Sweet Flavors

We make other sweet flavors in the theater style popper using a similar technique to how we make kettle corn. Instead of plain sugar we use flavored sugars or Glaze Pop. This includes homemade sugars by mixing extracts and plain sugar together or with store bought flavored sugars. To make these we use a 2:1 ratio of kernels to flavored sugar. In our case, 6 oz of kernels, 3oz of sugar. We utilize corn oil when making sweet flavors in the kettle. We heat up the kettle, start the motor and once the kettle is up to temperature, we add kernels and oil. When the kernels begin to pop, we open the lid and add our flavored sugars, close the lid, and continue popping until it slows down again. We then dump our flavored popcorn out to enjoy.

The theater-style popcorn popper, whether it's a 6oz or a larger model, serves as a versatile tool for crafting popcorn in smaller batches. It allows for efficient popping with less oil, promoting both healthier and more economical popcorn production. The fundamental process involves heating the kettle, activating the stirring mechanism, adding the right ingredients, and popping until complete. Specific flavor profiles, from savory to buttery and sweet, can be achieved by adjusting the ingredients and ratios accordingly. Hopefully this has helped shed some light on utilizing the theater-style popper to create a variety of mouthwatering popcorn delights.

Carmelizer

We utilized a carmelizer quite a bit when we had our popcorn shop. The carmelizer is terrific for adding a great flavorful candy coating onto popcorn. This isn't something you would use to make savory flavors and while you could probably make kettle corn in it, we never tried as we enjoyed making kettle corn the old-fashioned way. We are going to explain our process for flavors such as black cherry, apple, lemon, orange, grape, chocolate, strawberry, etc.

Our carmelizer is 5 gallons in size so our process will align to that. This will be easy to convert as most carmelizers you can buy are in 5-gallon increments.

We make our candy-coated popcorn in a carmelizer using a product called Basic Corn Treats Mix made by the Gold Medal Products company. The first thing we do is pop plain popcorn. Because we have a 5-gallon carmelizer, we pop 5 gallons of plain popcorn. We used butter coconut oil and kernels. We cannot stress this enough, when using a carmelizer it's important to use mushroom variety kernels as you need the heartiness of the popcorn. We make sure our popcorn to be completely cooled before using it. We turn the heat/motor switch on for our carmelizer and add 22oz of Basic Corn Treats Mix, they package them in hand single use packages or you can buy it in bulk and weigh it out. We then add 4 cups of white sugar and 12oz of water. We switch the motor on to stir up this mixture for about 30 seconds. Once that completes we add in a 4 oz stick of shortening and then put the lid on. Once the steam starts to show under the lid, we take it off and continue to cook the mixture. We are looking to get this up to a final temperature of 280 degrees. Just prior to that at 275 degrees we add ¼ cup of flavor mix. We use the Signature Blends flavorings that Gold Medal Products makes. It's a concentrated flavoring that works really well for candy coating. The one thing you want to remember is not to add the flavor mix too early in the process because it will burn off all the flavor leaving you with very bland popcorn.

We then turn off the heat/motor switch and turn the motor only switch on. While this is mixing, we dump in our 5 gallons of pre-popped popcorn. We let that mix for a few seconds and then tip the kettle to the mix position. We like to use a product called Free-N-Easy which helps the candy-coated corn not to stick. When the kettle is in the mix position, we spray in about 10 squirts of the Free-N-Easy and you'll notice the popcorn becomes less clumpy and starts to separate out. Once the popcorn was coated completely, we dumped it in a cooling tray and mixed it around using scoops. You'll notice that the coating on popcorn using a carmelizer is very uniform and candy looking.

The carmelizer played a pivotal role in our popcorn shop, allowing us to craft an array of candy-coated popcorn flavors that delighted customers. While it may not be suited for savory or kettle corn creations, its ability to transform plain popcorn into a mouthwatering candy-coated treat is undeniable.

Stove Top Popper

Popping popcorn on the stove is a great way to make some flavorful creations without the need for big machines and big batches. We are going to run through some techniques for a hand cranked popcorn popper that can be used on the stove. We prefer this stove top method because it's very similar to our other machines but uses a different heat source. There are a bunch of different hand crank poppers you can purchase with brands such as Whirley-Pop™, Great Northern, Time for Treats, Franklin's Original, Lehman's, and Cook N Home.

We use a 6-quart hand crank popper, and this is the process we follow. We add the following ingredients while the popper is not on the heat source, ½ cup popcorn kernels, 3 tablespoons butter coconut oil. We have an electric stove and we put the popper on the burner with the heat on medium-high heat. We then stir the popper slowly to keep the mixture moving until the popcorn popping slows down and then we remove it from the heat.

Savory Flavors

We utilize ½ cup of kernels and 3 tablespoons butter coconut oil to pop the popcorn completely following the usual method and afterwards while it's still hot, we put 1/8 of a cup of popcorn seasoning on it and stir to mix.

Butter Popcorn

For butter flavor we pop using ½ cup kernels, 3 tablespoons of butter coconut oil and ¾ teaspoon of Flavacol. We put this mixture on the stove and stir until the popping slows.

Kettle Corn

For kettle corn in the hand crank popcorn popper, we utilize ½ cup

kernels and 3 tablespoons corn oil. We put the mixture on the heat source and stir. When the kernels begin to pop, we then add 3 tablespoons of sugar. We continue popping until it slows and then add salt to taste afterwards.

Other Sweet Flavors

For other sweet flavors, very similar to kettle corn we put ½ cup kernels and 3 tablespoons of corn oil and then add to the heat. As it begins to pop we add ¼ cup of flavored sugar or glaze pop. We then continue to pop until the popping slows.

Chapter 16

More Popcorn Recipes

Kettle Corn

Kettle Popper

Ingredients:

- 1 ½ Cups Corn Oil
- 3 Cups Popcorn Kernels
- 1 ½ Cup Sugar

Instructions:

Add Oil and Popcorn to kettle and heat up. Once a few kernels start to pop, add the sugar. Continue to pop until finished. Add salt to taste.

Theater Popper (6oz Size)

Ingredients:

- 3oz corn oil
- 6oz Popcorn Kernels
- 3oz sugar

Instructions:

Add corn oil and popcorn kernels to kettle after preheating. Once popcorn begins to pop add sugar and continue popping until finished. Dump out and shake on salt. Cool popcorn while mixing.

Butter Flavor

Kettle Popper

Ingredients:

- 1 ½ Cups Butter Coconut Oil
- 3 Cups Popcorn Kernels (mushroom variety)
- 2 TBSP Flavacol

Instructions:

Add Oil, Popcorn, and Flavacol to kettle and heat up. Once the popcorn is fully popped dump and cool. You can always add more butter flavoring or melted clarified butter afterwards.

Theater Popper (6oz Size)

Ingredients:

- 2oz butter coconut oil
- 6oz Popcorn Kernels
- 1/2 Tablespoon Flavacol Use more for added saltiness and butter flavor.

Instructions:

Heat popcorn kettle. Add oil, kernels, and Flavacol. Pop until completed and dump.

Caramel Corn

Kettle Popper

Ingredients:

- 1 ½ Cups Butter Coconut Oil
- 3 Cups Popcorn Kernels
- 1 1/2 cups Gold Medal Caramel Glaze Pop

Instructions: Add oil and popcorn and heat. Once kernels start popping, add 1 1/2 cups Gold Medal Caramel Glaze Pop and stir until completely popped. Mix to cool.

Theater Popper (6oz Size)

Ingredients:

- 2oz Corn Oil
- 6oz Popcorn Kernels
- 3oz Gold Medal Caramel Glaze Pop

Instructions:

Add corn oil and popcorn kernels to kettle and heat. Once popcorn begins to pop add glaze pop and continue popping. Once popcorn slows, dump popcorn out of kettle.

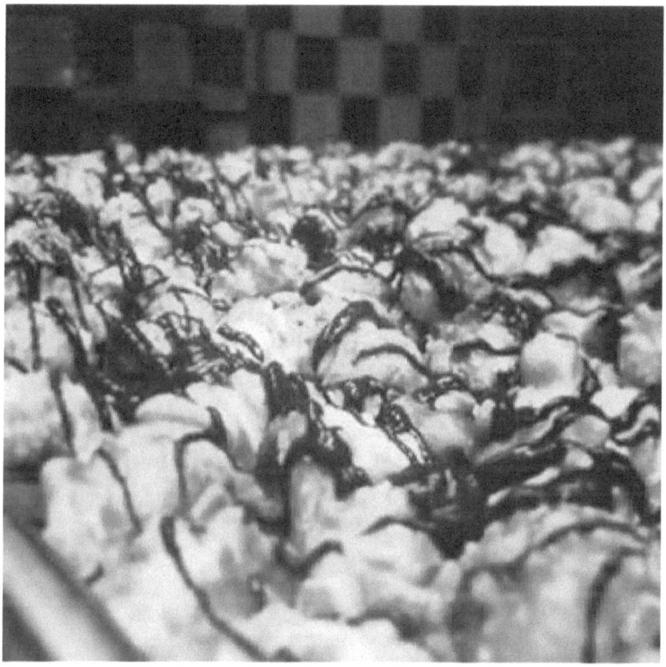

Chocolate Covered Caramel Corn

This is a start to some terrific popcorn flavors that you can make. Keep in mind that adding different toppings, chocolates, candies, and cereals can really kick your popcorn up a notch.

Hint: If you want your sugars (think plain sugar and floss sugars) to stick to your popcorn better, check out the Gold Medal Compound S product. Popping corn with this can really help.

Another thing that works great with making different flavor combinations is mixing flavors together as well. For example, ranch popcorn and white cheddar popcorn make a terrific cheesy ranch flavor. Mixing pink cherry and blue raspberry popcorn flavors together could make a great baby shower favor.

We've made sour popcorn as well by using a Gold Medal product called Sour Attitude. You sprinkle this on after the popcorn is fully popped like salt. It has a great sour flavor. Think of adding it to watermelon popcorn or blue raspberry for a sour candy flavor.

If you are interested in getting more recipes and also some video demonstrations on how to make flavored popcorn, check out www.popcorngenius.com/bookresources

Chapter 17

Conclusion

As we near the end of our journey through the captivating world of popcorn, it's time to reflect on the incredible voyage we've embarked upon. Popcorn is not just a snack; it's a testament to the enduring human spirit, a culinary marvel that transcends time and culture. Our exploration has taken us from the heartwarming stories of our families' connections to popcorn to the far reaches of its global impact, and it's clear that this humble kernel holds a special place in the hearts of people worldwide.

A Taste of Tradition

Popcorn is more than just a delicious treat; it's a link to our past, connecting us with generations of popcorn enthusiasts who found joy in its simplicity and deliciousness. From the earliest civilizations to modern-day moviegoers, the love for popcorn is a thread that weaves through the tapestry of human history. It's a reminder that some pleasures, like the satisfying crunch of a perfectly popped kernel, are truly timeless.

Our journey began with the origins of popcorn, tracing its humble beginnings to the ancient civilizations that reveled in its satisfying "pop." From the Aztecs to the Native Americans, popcorn was more than just sustenance; it was a symbol of celebration and togetherness. It's heartwarming to think that the joy we experience today when sharing popcorn with loved ones is a tradition that spans centuries.

Science: The Magic Behind the Pop

The science behind popcorn is a fascinating tale of chemical reactions and culinary magic. We delved into the intricate process that occurs when popcorn kernels are heated, transforming them from unassuming seeds into fluffy, edible delights. It's not just about the "pop" but also the anticipation, the excitement, and the sheer wonder of witnessing a simple kernel's transformation into something extraordinary.

Understanding the role of factors like kernel size, moisture content, and popping temperature has added a new layer of appreciation for the art of popping popcorn. The pursuit of the perfect pop is an endeavor that popcorn enthusiasts take to heart, tinkering with variables to achieve that ideal result. It's a testament to the dedication and passion that popcorn inspires in its devotees.

Popcorn's Versatility and Delight

But our journey doesn't stop at science. Popcorn's versatility is a testament to its enduring appeal. We've explored the countless ways that popcorn can be prepared and enjoyed. Whether you prefer the classic simplicity of buttered popcorn or crave the excitement of gourmet varieties infused with cheese, caramel, or exotic spices, there's a flavor to suit every palate.

Popcorn is a unifying force, bringing people together to share in the simple pleasure of a delicious snack. It's the companion of choice for movie nights, a staple at sporting events, and the star of cozy evenings at home. The aroma of freshly popped kernels creates an instant allure, drawing us in with its enticing scent. And the joy of biting into a perfectly popped kernel, experiencing that satisfying crunch and burst of flavor, is nothing short of pure bliss.

Popcorn: A Timeless Tradition

As we conclude our popcorn odyssey, it's clear that this beloved snack is more than just a passing fad. It's a timeless tradition that continues to bring delight and satisfaction to people of all walks of life. It's a reminder that the simple pleasures in life often hold the greatest value.

So, whether you're a casual snacker or a devoted popcorn enthusiast, there's always something new to learn and discover about this remarkable food. As you pop some corn and savor the many wonders of this beloved snack, remember that popcorn is not just a food; it's a celebration of tradition, a marvel of science, and a source of endless joy.

Whether you're sharing popcorn with loved ones, experimenting with new flavors, or simply enjoying the comforting familiarity of this humble yet extraordinary treat, remember that popcorn has the power to bring people together, spark conversations, create laughter, and forge cherished memories.

In the grand symphony of life, let popcorn be your tasty, crunchy note of happiness. Thank you for joining us on this popcorn-filled journey and may your love for this delightful snack continue to pop and flourish for generations to come.

If you want to continue your journey with us, be sure to check out www.popcorngenius.com/bookresources. So, remember, get out there and get poppin'.

Bibliography

1. Statista. "U.S. Households Consumption of Popcorn Products" [Online Data]. URL: https://www.statista.com/statistics/277153/us-households-consumption-of-popcorn-products/. Accessed 4 May 2023.

2. U.S. Census Bureau. "Popcorn Day" [Online Article]. URL: https://www.census.gov/newsroom/stories/popcorn-day.html. Accessed 4 May 2023.

3. National Confectioners Association. "Popcorn Market to Reach $18B Globally by 2031" [Online Article]. URL: https://candyusa.com/cst/popcorn-market-to-reach-18b-globally-by-2031/. Accessed 4 May 2023.

4. DriveInTheater.com. "History of Drive-In Theaters" [Online Article]. URL: https://www.driveintheater.com/drivhis1.htm. Accessed 6 May 2023.

5. Leelalicious. "Popcorn Flavours Around the World" [Online Article]. URL: https://leelalicious.com/popcorn-flavours-around-world/. Accessed 16 June 2023.

6. Taste for Cooking. "Unique Popcorn Flavors from Around the World" [Online Article]. URL: https://www.tasteforcooking.com/appetizers/unique-popcorn-flavors-from-around-the-world/. Accessed 4 May 2023.

7. Uncle Didi. "10 Trendiest or Weirdest Popcorn Flavours Around the World" [Online Article]. URL: https://www.uncledidi.com/10-trendiest-or-weirdest-popcorn-flavours-around-the-world/?utm_source=rss&utm_medium=rss&utm_campaign=10-trendiest-or-weirdest-popcorn-flavours-around-the-world. Accessed 6 May 2023

8. Verbnow. "Types of Popcorn Makers" [Online Article]. URL: https://verbnow.com/types-of-popcorn-makers/. Accessed 6 May 2023

9. AllRecipes. "Kettle Corn" [Online Recipe]. URL: https://www.allrecipes.com/recipe/20808/kettle-corn/. Accessed 16 June 2023.

10. My Baking Addiction. "Popcorn Balls" [Online Recipe]. URL: https://www.mybakingaddiction.com/popcorn-balls/. Accessed 16 June 2023.

11. Just a Mum NZ. "Maple Syrup Popcorn" [Online Recipe]. URL: https://justamumnz.com/2021/05/27/maple-syrup-popcorn/. Accessed 6 May 2023.

12. Culinary Ginger. "Mexican Popcorn" [Online Recipe]. URL: https://culinaryginger.com/mexican-popcorn/. Accessed 19 June 2023.

13. McCormick. "Chile Lime Popcorn" [Online Recipe]. URL: https://www.mccormick.com/recipes/appetizer/chile-lime-popcorn. Accessed 6 May 2023.

14. The Hungary Buddha. "Brazilian Pipoca" [Online Recipe]. URL: https://thehungarybuddha.com/2015/04/30/brazilian-pipoca/. Accessed 23 June 2023.

15. Flavors of Brazil. "Snacks: Popcorn (Pipoca)" [Online Article]. URL: http://flavorsofbrazil.blogspot.com/2012/03/snacks-popcorn-pipoca.html. Accessed 16 June 2023.

16. Food Network. "Canchita: The Un-Popped Popcorn of Peru" [Online Recipe]. URL: https://www.foodnetwork.com/recipes/ingrid-hoffmann/canchita-the-un-popped-popcorn-of-peru-recipe-1940701. Accessed 16 June 2023.

17. Olive Magazine. "Popcorn Ceviche" [Online Recipe]. URL: https://www.olivemagazine.com/recipes/fish-and-seafood/popcorn-ceviche/. Accessed 16 June 2023.

18. SBS Food. "Chimichurri Popcorn" [Online Recipe]. URL: https://www.sbs.com.au/food/recipes/chimichurri-popcorn. Accessed 6 May 2023.

19. Nestlé La Lechera. "Dulce de Leche Popcorn" [Online Recipe]. URL: https://www.goodnes.com/la-lechera/recipes/dulce-de-leche-popcorn/. Accessed [Insert Access Date].

20. My Colombian Recipes. "Mazorca Desgranada (Corn Kernels Snack)" [Online Recipe]. URL: https://www.mycolombianrecipes.com/mazorca-desgranada-corn-kernels-snack/. Accessed 2 July 2023.

21. YouTube - J.Kenji López-Alt. "How to Make Popcorn - The Science of Popcorn - Food Lab" [Online Video]. URL: https://www.youtube.com/watch?v=JZlli2J3ugs&embeds_euri=https%3A%2F%2Fwww.pinterest.ph%2F&source_ve_path=MjM4NTE&feature=emb_title&ab_channel=J.KenjiL%C3%B3pez-Alt. Accessed 6 May 2023.

22. Macheesmo. "Five Spice Popcorn" [Online Recipe]. URL: https://www.macheesmo.com/five-spice-popcorn/. Accessed 6 May 2023.

23. Lee Kum Kee USA. "Chiu Chow Chili Oil Popcorn" [Online Recipe]. URL: https://usa.lkk.com/en/recipes/chiu-chow-chili-oil-popcorn. Accessed 2 July 2023.

24. Times of India. "Masala Popcorn" [Online Recipe]. URL: https://recipes.timesofindia.com/recipes/masala-popcorn/rs62859671.cms. Accessed 2 July 2023.

25. V's Spice Route. "Tandoori Flavored Popcorn" [Online Recipe]. URL: https://vspiceroute.com/tandoori-flavored-popcorn/#:~:text=Instructions,and%20let%20the%20corn%20pop. Accessed 2 July 2023.

26. Nish Kitchen. "Jaggery Popcorn" [Online Recipe]. URL: https://nishkitchen.com/jaggery-popcorn-video/. Accessed 6 May 2023.

27. Food Republic. "Furikake Popcorn Recipe" [Online Recipe]. URL: https://www.foodrepublic.com/recipes/furikake-popcorn-recipe/. Accessed 2 June 2023.

28. DVCShop. "A Brief History of Disney Popcorn Buckets" [Online Article]. URL: https://dvcshop.com/a-brief-history-of-disney-popcorn-buckets/. Accessed 30 June 2023.

29. Saveur. "Savory Kimchi Nori Popcorn" [Online Recipe]. URL: https://www.saveur.com/article/Recipes/Savory-Kimchi-Nori-Popcorn/. Accessed 2 June 2023.

30. Serious Eats. "Thai Red Coconut Curry Flavored Popcorn" [Online Recipe]. URL: https://www.seriouseats.com/thai-red-coconut-curry-flavored-popcorn. Accessed 30 June 2023.

31. Naturally Ella. "Coconut Curry Popcorn" [Online Recipe]. URL: https://naturallyella.com/coconut-curry-popcorn/. Accessed 2 June 2023. Accessed 7 May 2023.

32. Flavour of the Diaspora. "Salt 'n Suya Popcorn" [Online Recipe]. URL: https://flavourofthediaspora.wordpress.com/2015/09/10/10-salt-n-suya-popcorn/. Accessed 6 May 2023.

33. Yummy Medley. "Popcorn and Peanuts" [Online Recipe]. URL: https://www.yummymedley.com/popcorn-and-peanuts/. Accessed 2 June 2023.

34. Taste. "Buttered Popcorn Flavored with Biltong and Peanut Brittle" [Online Recipe]. URL: https://taste.co.za/recipes/buttered-popcorn-flavoured-with-biltong-and-peanut-brittle/. Accessed 30 June 2023.

35. KitKat Group. "Popcorn Snack Mix" [Online Recipe]. URL: https://kitkatgroup.com/Shop/Product/142382C. Accessed 10 May 2023.

36. Always Order Dessert. "Ras el Hanout Spiced Popcorn with Chocolate and Pistachios" [Online Recipe]. URL: http://www.alwaysorderdessert.com/2014/01/ras-el-hanout-spiced-popcorn-with.html. Accessed 6 May 2023.

37. Joy the Baker. "Cinnamon Harissa Caramel Corn" [Online Recipe]. URL: https://joythebaker.com/2018/07/cinnamon-harissa-caramel-corn/. Accessed 30 June 2023.

38. Vegemite. "Vegemite Halloween Popcorn" [Online Recipe]. URL: https://vegemite.com.au/recipe/vegemite-halloween-popcorn/#newsletter. Accessed 6 May 2023.

39. New Zealand Woman's Weekly Food. "Peanut Butter Toffee Popcorn Lamingtons" [Online Recipe]. URL: https://www.nzwomansweeklyfood.co.nz/recipes/peanut-butter-toffee-popcorn-lamingtons-6970. Accessed 2 July 2023.

40. Fundraising Zone. "Caramel Corn Hokey Pokey Fundraising" [Online Article]. URL: https://fundraisingzone.com/brochure-fundraising-ideas/caramel-corn-hokey-pokey-fundraising/. Accessed 2 July 2023.

41. ShopPRI.com. "Manuka Honey Popcorn" [Online Recipe]. URL: https://www.shoppri.com/blogs/recipes/116602500-manuka-honey-popcorn. Accessed 2 June 2023.

42. BigOven. "Saffron Buttered Popcorn Recipe" [Online Recipe]. URL: https://www.bigoven.com/recipe/saffron-buttered-popcorn/46817. Accessed 2 June 2023.

43. TrendHunter. "Popcorn Bark" [Online Article]. URL: https://www.trendhunter.com/trends/popcorn-bark. Accessed 6 May 2023.

44. UniQucorn. "Turkish Delight Popcorn" [Product Page]. URL: https://www.uniqucorn.com/product/turkish-delight/. Accessed 30 June 2023.

45. goop. "Olive Oil and Herb Popcorn" [Online Recipe]. URL: https://goop.com/recipes/olive-oil-and-herb-popcorn/. Accessed 2 June 2023.

46. Serious Eats. "Za'atar (Thyme, Sesame, Sumac) Spiced Popcorn" [Online Recipe]. URL: https://www.seriouseats.com/zaatar-thyme-sesame-sumac-spiced-popcorn-flavor-recipe. Accessed 30 June 2023.

47. Refinery29. "Chocolate Sesame Popcorn" [Online Recipe]. URL: https://www.refinery29.com/en-us/chocolate-sesame-popcorn-recipe-video. Accessed 30 June 2023.

48. The Steady Cook. "Popcorn with Sumac and Dill" [Online Recipe]. URL: https://thesteadycook.com/2020/11/06/popcorn-with-sumac-and-dill/. Accessed 30 June 2023.

49. Plant Based on a Budget. "Chai Spiced Popcorn" [Online Recipe]. URL: https://plantbasedonabudget.com/chai-spiced-popcorn/. Accessed 2 June 2023.

50. Verbnow. "Types of Popcorn Makers" [Online Article]. URL: https://verbnow.com/types-of-popcorn-makers/. Accessed 30 June 2023.

51. WebstaurantStore. "Types of Popcorn and Popcorn Machines" [Online Guide]. URL: https://www.webstaurantstore.com/guide/517/types-of-popcorn-and-popcorn-machines.html. Accessed 2 June 2023.

52. Home Stratosphere. "Types of Popcorn Makers" [Online Article]. URL: https://www.homestratosphere.com/types-of-popcorn-makers/. Accessed 2 July 2023.

53. Amazon.com. "Presto 04820 PopLite Hot Air Popper" [Online Product Page]. URL: https://www.amazon.com/Presto-04820-PopLite-Hot-Popper/dp/B00006IUWA?th=1. Accessed 2 July 2023.

54. GMPopcorn.com. "PopMaxx Value Popper 2552" [Online Product Page]. URL: https://shop.gmpopcorn.com/products/popmaxx-value-popper-2552. Accessed 30 June 2023.

55. Lékué. "Popcorn Maker" [Online Product Page]. URL: https://www.lekue.com/us/popcorn-lekue. Accessed 2 July 2023.

56. Nordic Ware. "Microwave Popcorn Popper" [Online Product Page]. URL: https://www.nordicware.com/products/microwave-popcorn-popper/. Accessed 30 June 2023.

57. West Bend. "Stir Crazy Popcorn Popper" [Online Product Page]. URL: https://westbend.com/collections/stir-crazy/products/stir-crazy. Accessed 2 July 2023.

58. Amazon.com. "Nostalgia RKP630 2.5-Ounce Kettle Popcorn Maker" [Online Product Page]. URL: https://www.amazon.com/Nostalgia-RKP630-2-5-Ounce-Kettle-Popcorn/dp/B0016NUYCO. Accessed 2 July 2023.

59. Paragon Concessions. "Paragon Theater Pop 4-Ounce Popcorn Machine" [Online Product Page]. URL: https://www.paragonconcessions.com/products/paragon-theater-pop-4-ounce-popcorn-machine?gclid=Cj0KCQjwr82iBhCuARIsAO0EAZxHyK8iSp2mB86pkmWAM0nNQhz9lXlim9dx6eTcQbaWwBRZsK4_OgEaAjQ7EALw_wcB. Accessed 2 July 2023.

60. WhirleyPopShop.com. "Whirley Pop Stovetop Popcorn Popper" [Online Product Page]. URL: https://www.whirleypopshop.com/. Accessed 2 June 2023.

61. Pie Iron. "Old-Fashioned Popcorn Popper Original by Rome" [Online Product Page]. URL: https://www.pieiron.com/products/old-fashioned-popcorn-popper-original-by-rome. Accessed 2 July 2023.

62. DVCShop. "A Brief History of Disney Popcorn Buckets" [Online Article]. URL: https://dvcshop.com/a-brief-history-of-disney-popcorn-buckets/. Accessed 4 May 2023.

63. Leealicious. "Popcorn Flavours Around the World" [Online Article]. URL: https://leelalicious.com/popcorn-flavours-around-world/. Accessed 3 June 2023.

64. Amish Country Popcorn. "Popcorn's Rise to Popularity" [Online Article]. URL: https://amishcountrypopcorn.com/blog/popcorns-rise-to-popularity/. Accessed 4 May 2023.

65. Times of India. "The History of Popcorn: How This One Food Changed the Snacking Option World Over" [Online Article]. URL: https://timesofindia.indiatimes.com/life-style/food-news/the-history-of-popcorns-how-this-one-food-changed-the-snacking-option-world-over/articleshow/77769799.cms. Accessed 2 June 2023.

66. FoodNavigator. "Culture Pop Blends French Gastronomy and Healthy On-The-Go Popcorn" [Online Article]. URL: https://www.foodnavigator.com/Article/2017/04/11/Culture-Pop-blends-French-gastronomy-and-healthy-on-the-go-popcorn. Accessed 4 May 2023.

67. LinkedIn. "The Curious Case of Milk Popcorn in Nigeria" [Online Article]. URL: https://www.linkedin.com/pulse/curious-case-milk-popcorn-nigeria-ahmed-bulbulia. Accessed 30 June 2023.

68. Ada's Recipes. "Nigerian Popcorn Recipe: It's Homemade and Tasty" [Online Recipe]. URL: https://www.adasrecipes.com/nigerian-popcorn-recipe-its-homemade-and-tasty/#:~:text=Nigerian%20popcorn%20recipe%20is%20a,moi%20moi%2C%20corn%20and%20ukwa. Accessed 4 May 2023.

69. Medium. "Foods Americans Eat That Seem Strange to the French" [Online Article]. URL: https://medium.com/illumination/foods-americans-eat-that-seem-strange-to-the-french-d32696c17a61. Accessed 1 June 2023.

70. Flavors of Brazil. "Snacks: Popcorn (Pipoca)" [Online Article]. URL: http://flavorsofbrazil.blogspot.com/2012/03/snacks-popcorn-pipoca.html. Accessed 2 June 2023.

71. Penn State University. "How Microwave Popcorn Works" [Online Article]. URL: https://sites.psu.edu/siowfa15/2015/09/17/how-microwave-popcorn-works/#:~:text=Microwavable%20popcorn%20bags%20work%20the,will%20pop%20right%20into%20them. Accessed 2 June 2023.

72. Wikipedia. "Microwave Popcorn" [Online Article]. URL: https://en.wikipedia.org/wiki/Microwave_popcorn. Accessed 2 July 2023. Accessed 4 May 2023.

73. YouTube - ACS Webinars. "How Microwave Popcorn Pops" [Online Video]. URL: https://www.youtube.com/watch?v=NtwkzXi6ylc&ab_channel=ACSWebinars. Accessed 4 May 2023.

74. Baked Bree. "Perfect Stovetop Popcorn" [Online Recipe]. URL: https://bakedbree.com/perfect-stovetop-popcorn. Accessed 28 June 2023.

75. Simply Recipes. "Perfect Popcorn" [Online Recipe]. URL: https://www.simplyrecipes.com/recipes/perfect_popcorn/. Accessed 4 May 2023.

76. Amy's Healthy Baking. "Stovetop Air-Popped Popcorn" [Online Recipe]. URL: https://amyshealthybaking.com/blog/2018/03/18/stovetop-air-popped-popcorn/. Accessed 4 May 2023.

77. Wholefully. "Movie Theatre Popcorn at Home" [Online Recipe]. URL: https://wholefully.com/movie-theatre-popcorn-home/. Accessed 28 June 2023.

78. Dwell by Michelle. "Best Home Theater Popcorn Machines" [Online Article]. URL: https://dwellbymichelle.com/best-home-theater-popcorn-machines/. Accessed 2 July 2023.

79. Food Network. "Best Popcorn Machines" [Online Article]. URL: https://www.foodnetwork.com/how-to/packages/shopping/product-reviews/best-popcorn-machines. Accessed 4 May 2023.

80. Serious Eats. "How to Make Popcorn the Best Way" [Online Article]. URL: https://www.seriouseats.com/how-to-make-popcorn-best-way#:~:text=The%20air%20popper%20works%20by,of%20six%20minutes%20per%20batch. Accessed 4 May 2023.

81. Delighted Cooking. "What Is an Air Popper?" [Online Article]. URL: https://www.delightedcooking.com/what-is-an-air-popper.htm. Accessed 30 June 2023.

82. YouTube - RICHARD IN THE KITCHEN. "How to Make Perfect Popcorn on the Stove" [Online Video]. URL: https://www.youtube.com/watch?v=L2VINOt4OW4&ab_channel=RICHARDINTHEKITCHEN. Accessed 28 June 2023.

83. The Cookful. "15 Ways to Pop Popcorn" [Online Article]. URL: https://thecookful.com/15-ways-pop-popcorn/. Accessed 4 May 2023.

84. Popcorn Board. "History of Popcorn" [Online Article]. URL: https://www.popcorn.org/All-About-Popcorn/History-of-Popcorn. Accessed 28 June 2023.

85. Serious Eats. "The History of Popcorn in Movie Theaters" [Online Article]. URL: https://www.seriouseats.com/popcorn-history-movie-theaters. Accessed 28 June 2023.

86. History. "A History of Popcorn" [Online Article]. URL: https://www.history.com/news/a-history-of-popcorn. Accessed 28 June 2023.

87. PBS Food. "The History of Popcorn" [Online Article]. URL: https://www.pbs.org/food/the-history-kitchen/popcorn-history/. Accessed 4 May 2023.

88. Popcorn for the People. "The History of Popcorn" [Online Article]. URL: https://www.popcornforthepeople.com/blogs/blog/the-history-of-popcorn. Accessed 2 July 2023.

89. History of Fast Food. "History of Popcorn" [Online Article]. URL: http://www.historyoffastfood.com/fast-food-types/history-of-popcorn/. Accessed 4 May 2023.

90. America's Favorite Popcorn. "Fun Facts About Popcorn" [Online Article]. URL: https://americasfavoritepopcorn.com/blogs/all-blogs/fun-facts-about-popcorn. Accessed 2 July 2023.

91. Popcorn Festival. "Valparaiso Popcorn Festival" [Online Event Page]. URL: https://www.popcornfestival.com/parade/. Accessed 28 June 2023.

92. Valparaiso Events. "Valparaiso Popcorn Festival" [Online Event Page]. URL: https://www.valparaisoevents.com/event/valparaiso-popcorn-festival. Accessed 2 July 2023.

93. Nerdist. "How Popcorn Became a Movie Theater Snack: The Full History" [Online Article]. URL: https://nerdist.com/article/how-popcorn-became-a-movie-theater-snack-full-history/. Accessed 8 July 2023.

94. USDA Agricultural Research Service. "Popcorn Explosion" [Online Article]. URL: https://www.nal.usda.gov/exhibits/speccoll/exhibits/show/popcorn/popcorn-explosion. Accessed 28 June 2023.

95. Youth Policy Review. "Buttered Popcorn Economic Indicators" [Online Article]. URL: https://www.youthpolicyreview.com/post/buttered-popcorn-economic-indicators. Accessed 2 July 2023.

96. Business Desk NZ. "It's a Popcorn Economy, and We're a B-Movie" [Online Article]. URL: https://businessdesk.co.nz/article/finance/its-a-popcorn-economy-and-were-a-b-movie. Accessed 28 June 2023.

97. Great Lakes Popcorn Company. "History of Popcorn" [Online Article]. URL: https://grpopcorn.com/blogs/news/history-of-popcorn. Accessed 2 July 2023.

98. Reist Popcorn. "Pop Culture" [Online Article]. URL: https://www.reistpopcorn.com/pop-culture/. Accessed 8 July 2023.

99. Érudit. "The Economic Significance of Popcorn" [Online Article]. URL: https://id.erudit.org/iderudit/013351ar. Accessed 2 July 2023.

100. IMDb. "The Late Shift (TV Movie 1996)" [Online Movie Page]. URL: https://www.imdb.com/title/tt0117571/characters/nm0000106#:~:text=Phone%20Voice%20%3A%20I%20only%20eat,ready%20to%20watch%20a%20video. Accessed 8 July 2023.

101. America's Favorite Popcorn. "Evolution of Popcorn Poppers" [Online Article]. URL: https://americasfavoritepopcorn.com/blogs/all-blogs/evolution-of-popcorn-poppers#:~:text=Some%20individuals%20attempted%20to%20cook,from%20Illinois%20named%20Charles%20Cretors. Accessed 28 June 2023.

102. PopMaize. "Popcorn Popper History" [Online Article]. URL: https://popmaize.com/popcorn-popper-history/. Accessed 8 July 2023.

103. Popcorn Boss. "Microwave Popcorn History" [Online Article]. URL: https://www.popcornboss.com/microwave-popcorn-history.html#:~:text=As%20the%20story%20is%20reported,by%20it%20and%20they%20popped. Accessed 28 June 2023.

104.McClain Popcorn. "The Complete and Updated History of Popcorn" [Online Article]. URL: https://www.mcclainpopcorn.com/popcorn-history/the-complete-and-updated-history-of-popcorn/#:~:text=Charles%20Cretors%20created%20a%20portable,popper%20eight%20years%20later. Accessed 28 June 2023.

105.U.S. Food and Drug Administration (FDA). "Science and History of GMOs and Other Food Modification Processes" [Online Article]. URL: https://www.fda.gov/food/agricultural-biotechnology/science-and-history-gmos-and-other-food-modification-processes. Accessed 8 July 2023.

106.Food for Net. "Best Oil for Popping Popcorn" [Online Article]. URL: https://foodfornet.com/best-oil-for-popping-popcorn/. Accessed 2 July 2023.

107.Smokin' Joes RI Branch. "Best Oil for Popcorn" [Online Article]. URL: https://www.smokinjoesribranch.com/best-oil-for-popcorn/. Accessed 8 July 2023.

108.Chef's Pencil. "Best Oil for Popcorn" [Online Article]. URL: https://www.chefspencil.com/best-oil-for-popcorn/. Accessed 2 July 2023.

109.USDA Agricultural Research Service. "How Does Popcorn Pop?" [Online Article]. URL: https://www.nal.usda.gov/exhibits/speccoll/exhibits/show/popcorn/how-does-popcorn-pop-#:~:text=As%20the%20kernel%20heats%20up,turning%20the%20kernel%20inside%20out. Accessed 2 July 2023.

110.Scientific American. "Explore the 'Pop' in Popcorn" [Online Article]. URL: https://www.scientificamerican.com/article/explore-the-pop-in-popcorn/. Accessed 2 July 2023.

111.Carolina Science and Math Education Network. "The Science of Popcorn" [Online Article]. URL: https://knowledge.carolina.com/discipline/physical-science/the-science-of-popcorn/. Accessed 8 July 2023.

112.Our Everyday Life. "How Popcorn Storage Affects Popping" [Online Article]. URL: https://oureverydaylife.com/how-popcorn-storage-affects-popping-12397841.html. Accessed 8 July 2023.

113.America's Favorite Popcorn. "Why Do Some Popcorn Kernels Not Pop?" [Online Article]. URL: https://americasfavoritepopcorn.com/blogs/all-blogs/why-do-some-popcorn-kernels-not-pop#:~:text=Popcorn%20kernels%20will%20not%20pop%20if%20they%20contain%20too%20little,popcorn%20kernel%20to%20not%20explode. Accessed 10 May 2023.

114.Verbnow. "Types of Popcorn Makers" [Online Article]. URL: https://verbnow.com/types-of-popcorn-makers/. Accessed 8 July 2023.

115.Gourmet Gift Baskets. "Where Does Popcorn Come From?" [Online Article]. URL: https://www.gourmetgiftbaskets.com/Blog/post/where-does-popcorn-come-from.aspx. Accessed 2 July 2023.

116.The Pioneer Woman. "Types of Popcorn" [Online Article]. URL: https://www.thepioneerwoman.com/food-cooking/cooking-tips-tutorials/a98090/types-of-popcorn/. Accessed 8 July 2023.

117.WebstaurantStore. "Types of Popcorn and Popcorn Machines" [Online Guide]. URL: https://www.webstaurantstore.com/guide/517/types-of-popcorn-and-popcorn-machines.html#:~:text=There%20are%20two%20types%20of,each%20a%20'best'%20use. Accessed 8 July 2023.

118.L'Academie. "Types of Popcorn" [Online Article]. URL: https://www.lacademie.com/types-of-popcorn/. Accessed 2 July 2023.

119.Popcornity. "51 Fun Facts About Popcorn" [Online Article]. URL: https://popcornity.com/51-fun-facts-about-popcorn/. Accessed 2 July 2023.

120. Atom Tickets. "National Popcorn Day Trivia: 30 Fun Facts" [Online Article]. URL: https://atomtickets.com/movie-news/national-popcorn-day-trivia-facts/. Accessed 10 May 2023.

121. Fact Retriever. "Popcorn Facts" [Online Article]. URL: https://www.factretriever.com/popcorn-facts. Accessed 10 May 2023.

122. Popcorn Board. "Corny Facts" [Online Article]. URL: https://www.popcorn.org/All-About-Popcorn/Corny-Facts. Accessed 10 May 2023.

123. Popcorn Boss. "Popcorn Facts" [Online Article]. URL: https://www.popcornboss.com/popcorn-facts.html. Accessed 10 May 2023.

124. WebMD. "Health Benefits of Popcorn" [Online Article]. URL: https://www.webmd.com/food-recipes/health-benefits-popcorn#:~:text=There%20are%20a%20few%20health,disease%2C%20and%20hypertension%20in%20humans. Accessed 10 May 2023.

125. One Good Thing by Jillee. "The Surprising Benefits of My Favorite Snack: Popcorn" [Online Article]. URL: https://www.onegoodthingbyjillee.com/the-surprising-benefits-of-my-favorite-snack-popcorn/. Accessed 9 May 2023.

126. American Heart Association. "Popcorn as a Snack: Healthy Hit or Dietary Horror Show?" [Online Article]. URL: https://www.heart.org/en/news/2019/06/18/popcorn-as-a-snack-healthy-hit-or-dietary-horror-show#:~:text=In%20addition%20to%20fiber%2C%20popcorn,popcorn%20is%20its%20high%20satiety. Accessed 9 May 2023.

127. Sephra USA. "Is Popcorn Good for You?" [Online Article]. URL: https://sephrausa.com/blogs/blog/is-popcorn-good-for-you/#:~:text=Protects%20against%20free%20radicals.,damage%20healthy%20cells%20and%20DNA. Accessed 9 May 2023.

128. Cleveland Clinic. "9 Best Tips to Help Make Healthier Popcorn" [Online Article]. URL: https://health.clevelandclinic.org/9-best-tips-help-make-healthier-popcorn/. Accessed 9 May 2023.

129.Men's Health. "Is Popcorn Healthy?" [Online Article]. URL: https://www.menshealth.com/nutrition/a41612848/is-popcorn-healthy/. Accessed 30 June 2023.

130.South Tampa Smiles. "Is Popcorn Bad for Your Teeth?" [Online Article]. URL: https://www.southtampasmiles.com/is-popcorn-bad-for-your-teeth/#:~:text=Popcorn%20is%20one%20of%20those,the%20debris%20and%20lactic%20acid. Accessed 11 May 2023.

131.Lybrate. "Benefits of Popcorn and Its Side Effects" [Online Article]. URL: https://www.lybrate.com/topic/benefits-of-popcorn-and-its-side-effects. Accessed 9 May 2023.

132.Medical News Today. "Is Popcorn a Healthy Snack?" [Online Article]. URL: https://www.medicalnewstoday.com/articles/324763#:~:text=Premade%20popcorn%20often%20contains%20a,make%20popcorn%20an%20unhealthful%20snack. Accessed 9 May 2023.

About the Authors: Kelli and Frank

Meet Kelli and Frank, a dynamic duo with a passion for popcorn that goes beyond mere snacking. Married for over 22 years, this husband-and-wife team shares their popcorn prowess with the world through their YouTube channel, Popcorn Genius.

With two sons, Luca and Frankie, who are the light of their lives, Kelli and Frank's journey into the popcorn industry is a story of love, family, and entrepreneurial spirit. Their adventure began one fateful night over dinner when a playful conversation sparked the idea of opening a gourmet popcorn shop. This dream quickly turned into reality as they embarked on a journey filled with research, excitement, and a dash of serendipity.

Their venture, The Magic Kernel, became more than just a shop; it was a testament to their creativity and dedication. From drawing up plans to acquiring a treasure trove of equipment from a classified ad, Kelli and Frank poured their hearts into making their vision come to life. Their commitment to quality and innovation was evident in their carefully crafted recipes and the wide array of flavors they offered, from classic caramel corn to inventive combinations like pizza and ranch popcorn.

Despite the challenges and long hours, the joy of seeing customers smile and the sense of community that formed around their shop made every effort worthwhile. However, life has its twists and turns, and the couple made the difficult decision to close their shop temporarily to focus on family. Yet, their passion for popcorn never waned.

Today, Kelli and Frank continue to spread their love for popcorn through The Popcorn Genius, teaching others how to create delicious popcorn from the comfort of their own homes. Their story is a reminder that with love, creativity, and a little bit of popcorn, anything is possible.

To learn more, and to follow Kelli & Frank visit popcorngenius.com

Made in United States
Troutdale, OR
11/03/2026

56852697R00096